ADVANCES IN

Anesthesia

Editor-in-Chief
Thomas M. McLoughlin, MD

ELSEVIER

An Imprint of Elsevier, Inc.

PHILADELPHIA LONDON TORONTO MONTREAL SYDNEY TOKYO

VOLUMES 1 THROUGH 26 (OUT OF PRINT)

VOLUME 27

Anesthetic Management of Interventional Neuroradiological Procedures, *by Shailendra Joshi, Sean D. Lavine, and William L. Young*

Perioperative Management of the Opioid-Tolerant Patient, *by Christopher Viscomi and Jared K. Pearson*

Preoperative Stress Syndromes and Their Evaluation, Consultation, and Management, *by Edward R. Norris, Muhamad Aly Rifai, and Michael W. Kaufmann*

Genomics: Implications for Anesthesia, Perioperative Care and Outcomes, *by Simon C. Body*

Retirement Planning for Physicians, *by J. Bruce Levis Jr and David S. Markle*

Nonopioid Adjuvants in Multimodal Therapy for Acute Perioperative Pain, *by Bryan S. Williams and Asokumar Buvanendran*

Evidence-Based Update and Controversies in the Treatment and Prevention of Postoperative Nausea and Vomiting, *by Ashraf S. Habib and Tong J. Gan*

Impact of Central Neuraxial Analgesia on the Progress of Labor, *by Christopher R. Cambic and Cynthia A. Wong*

Regional Anesthesia in Trauma, *by Laura Clark and Marina Varbanova*

VOLUME 28

Herbal Supplements and Nutraceuticals: Perioperative Considerations, *by Maunak V. Rana and Gregory N. Kozlov*

Modern Understanding of Intraoperative Mechanical Ventilation in Normal and Diseased Lungs, *by Ralph Gertler and Girish P. Joshi*

VOLUME 29

Drug Diversion, Chemical Dependence, and Anesthesiology, *by John E. Tetzlaff*

Anesthesia for Intrauterine Fetal Therapy and Ex Utero Intrapartum Therapy, *by Kha M. Tran*

Clinical Pathways for Total Joint Arthroplasty: Essential Components for Success, *by Rebecca L. Johnson, Christopher M. Duncan, and James R. Hebl*

Vice President, Continuity Publishing: Kimberly Murphy
Editor: Yonah Korngold

Reprints: For copies of 100 or more of articles in this publication, please contact the Commercial Reprints Department, Elsevier Inc., 360 Park Avenue South, New York, NY 10010-1710. Tel: (212) 633-3812; Fax: (212) 462-1935; E-mail: reprints@elsevier.com.

Printed in the United States of America.

Editorial Office:
Elsevier
1600 John F. Kennedy Blvd,
Suite 1800
Philadelphia, PA 19103-2899

International Standard Serial Number: 0737-6146
International Standard Book Number-13: 978-0-323-08870-1

ADVANCES IN
Anesthesia

ADVANCES IN Anesthesia

CONTRIBUTORS

SASCHA BEUTLER, MD, PhD, Assistant Professor, Department of Anesthesiology, Perioperative and Pain Medicine, Brigham and Women's Hospital, Boston, Massachusetts

ANDRE M. DE WOLF, MD, Professor, Department of Anesthesiology, Feinberg School of Medicine, Northwestern University, Chicago, Illinois

MATTHEW B. FRIESE, MD, PhD, Resident, Department of Anesthesiology, Perioperative and Pain Medicine, Brigham and Women's Hospital, Boston, Massachusetts

NATHANIEL H. GREENE, MD, Academic Chief Resident and Bonica Scholar, Department of Anesthesiology and Pain Medicine, University of Washington, Seattle, Washington

NEIL A. HANSON, MD, Virginia Mason Medical Center, Seattle, Washington

JAN F.A. HENDRICKX, MD, PhD, Staff Anesthesiologist, Department of Anesthesiology/CCM, OLV Hospital, Aalst, Belgium

ANTHONY G. HUDETZ, DBM, PhD, Professor, Departments of Anesthesiology, Physiology, and Biophysics, Medical College of Wisconsin, Milwaukee, Wisconsin

ALAIN F. KALMAR, MD, PhD, Staff Anesthesiologist, Department of Anesthesiology, University Medical Center Groningen, University of Groningen, Groningen, The Netherlands

LORETTA KOWALICK, RN, CMM, Allentown Anesthesia Associates, Allentown, Pennsylvania

LORRI A. LEE, MD, Professor, Department of Anesthesiology and Pain Medicine; Adjunct, Department of Neurological Surgery, University of Washington, Seattle, Washington

GEORGE A. MASHOUR, MD, PhD, Assistant Professor, Departments of Anesthesiology and Neurosurgery, University of Michigan Medical School, Ann Arbor, Michigan

MARIA D. MOTOVIDLAK-THOMAS, CRNA, BA, MSN, Lehigh Valley Anesthesia Services, Lehigh Valley Health Network, Allentown, Pennsylvania

MICHAEL F. MULROY, MD, Faculty Anesthesiologist, Virginia Mason Medical Center, Seattle, Washington

JUHAN PAISTE, MD, MBA, Allentown Anesthesia Associates; Department of Anesthesiology, Lehigh Valley Health Network, Allentown, Pennsylvania

IVAN J. PERRY, DO, Allentown Anesthesia Associates; Department of Anesthesiology, Lehigh Valley Health Network, Allentown, Pennsylvania

RYAN P. PONG, MD, Anesthesiology Faculty, Department of Anesthesiology, Virginia Mason Medical Center, Seattle, Washington

CHRISTOPHER M. REIDY, MD, Assistant Professor, Department of Anesthesiology, University of Wisconsin Hospital and Clinics, University of Wisconsin-Madison, Madison, Wisconsin

AMOD SAWARDEKAR, MD, Department of Pediatric Anesthesiology, Ann & Robert H. Lurie Children's Hospital of Chicago, Assistant Professor of Anesthesiology, Feinberg School of Medicine, Northwestern University, Chicago, Illinois

RAVI SHAH, MD, Department of Pediatric Anesthesiology, Ann & Robert H. Lurie Children's Hospital of Chicago, Assistant Professor of Anesthesiology, Feinberg School of Medicine, Northwestern University, Chicago, Illinois

BRIAN D. SITES, MD, Associate Professor of Anesthesiology and Orthopedic Surgery, Director of Orthopedic and Regional Anesthesiology, Departments of Anesthesiology and Pain Management, Dartmouth-Hitchcock Medical Center, Lebanon, New Hampshire

SANTHANAM SURESH, MD, FAAP, Department of Pediatric Anesthesiology, Ann & Robert H. Lurie Children's Hospital of Chicago, Professor of Anesthesiology & Pediatrics, Feinberg School of Medicine, Northwestern University, Chicago, Illinois

MAGNUS K. TEIG, BSc (Hon), MBChB, MRCP, FRCA, Lecturer-Fellow in Neuroanesthesiology, Department of Anesthesiology, University of Michigan Medical School, Ann Arbor, Michigan

CONTENTS VOLUME 30 • 2012

Advances in Anesthesia 30 (2012) 1–12

ADVANCES IN ANESTHESIA

An Update on Postoperative Delirium

Matthew B. Friese, MD, PhD, Sascha Beutler, MD, PhD*

Department of Anesthesiology, Perioperative and Pain Medicine, Brigham and Women's Hospital, 75 Francis Street, CWN L1, Boston, MA 02115, USA

Keywords

• Postoperative • Delirium • Elderly • Anesthesiology • Risk factors • Prevention

Key Points

- Postoperative delirium is a change in cognition that occurs frequently during the postoperative period, particularly in the elderly.
- Postoperative delirium is a major public health concern that negatively affects morbidity and mortality and places a large fiscal burden on the health care system.
- Although the anesthesiologist's care of these patients has often ended well before the symptoms of postoperative delirium begin, they can play an important role in the prevention of this disease.

The *Diagnostic and Statistical Manual of Mental Disorders* (Fourth Edition, Text Revision) defines delirium as a change in cognition that is characterized by an acute onset of inattention and either disorganized thinking or a change in the level of consciousness [1]. Delirium in the postoperative period is common, affecting more than 50% of patients in certain surgical settings. However, many anesthesiologists are unaware of its high prevalence, because postoperative delirium often manifests days after the surgery [2–4]. Anesthesiologists routinely administer powerful medications during the perioperative period that can play a key role in the cause of postoperative delirium [4–6]. This article provides a review of delirium, with a special focus on the role that anesthesiologists play in its prevention, diagnosis, and treatment.

PREVALENCE

Although postoperative delirium may occur in almost any patient, certain populations are at a higher risk. The elderly are particularly prone to postoperative delirium; for each year over the age of 65 years, the risk of developing delirium increases by 2% [2,7]. The preexistence of cognitive impairment in an elderly patient, even if subtle, increases a patient's risk for developing delirium.

Disclosures: None.

*Corresponding author. *E-mail address:* Sbeutler@partners.org

0737-6146/12/$ – see front matter
http://dx.doi.org/10.1016/j.aan.2012.06.002

A prospective study evaluating preoperative and postoperative neuropsychological performance in patients older than 70 years without baseline delirium found that those who developed postoperative delirium had significantly slower mean reaction times and greater variability of reaction time during preoperative testing [8].

Delirium is especially prevalent in the intensive care unit (ICU) setting, where it has been detected in more than 83% of mechanically ventilated patients and in 70% of all patients older than 65 [9,10]. Although young patients have a decreased risk compared with the elderly, the prevalence of ICU delirium in patients younger than 65 years is still 57% [11].

RISK FACTORS

Several other nonmodifiable risk factors predispose patients to the development of postoperative delirium, including hypertension, smoking history; alcohol history, visual/hearing impairment, depression, and preexisting cognitive impairment (Box 1). Other factors inherent to underlying illness are difficult to influence. For instance, increasing severity of illness, as determined by the Acute Physiology and Chronic Health Evaluation II (APACHE II) score, is associated with delirium [11]. Other disease factors associated with delirium include acidosis, anemia, fever/infection/sepsis, hypotension, metabolic disturbances

Box 1: Overview of common risk factors for delirium

Patient factors

Age (2% increase in prevalence for each year over 65 years of age)
Preexisting cognitive impairment or depression
History of hypertension
Vascular disease/history of stroke
History of alcohol abuse, substance abuse, or smoking
Visual or hearing impairment

Illness factors

Metabolic derangements
Anemia, fever/infection/sepsis, or hypotension
Elevated APACHE II score

Environmental and iatrogenic factors

Use of medications (especially benzodiazepines, opioids, and anticholinergics)
Hypoxia
Presence of intravenous lines, bladder catheters, and/or physical restraints
Sleep disturbances
Withholding visual or hearing aids

(derangements in sodium, calcium, and blood urea nitrogen), and respiratory disease [12,13].

The modifiable risks factors are often iatrogenic and environmental in nature. Exposure to certain medications, including benzodiazepines and opioids, is often implicated in the development of postoperative delirium [12]. The role that opioids play in the development of delirium is complicated; for instance, poorly controlled pain is associated with a high risk of delirium, but treatment with opioids, most notably meperidine, is also associated with a high risk [7,14]. Immobilization of patients because of catheters and restraints occurs frequently in the hospital setting and can contribute to the development of delirium. Sleep disturbance is a pervasive problem in all hospitalized patients and is particularly common in patients in the ICU. In general, critically ill patients are the patient group exposed to the greatest numbers of risk factors for development of delirium. One study found that patients in the medical ICU had an average of 11 risk factors for delirium per patient, likely contributing to its high prevalence [15].

MORBIDITY AND MORTALITY ARE INCREASED IN PATIENTS WITH DELIRIUM

When corrected for age and medical comorbidities, patients with delirium have significantly higher morbidity and mortality than those without delirium (Fig. 1) [16]. One study showed that the inpatient mortality rate was 7% higher in patients with delirium compared with those without [17]. Moreover, the impact of delirium on patients and their families can be great, because patients who develop delirium are more likely to develop hospital-acquired

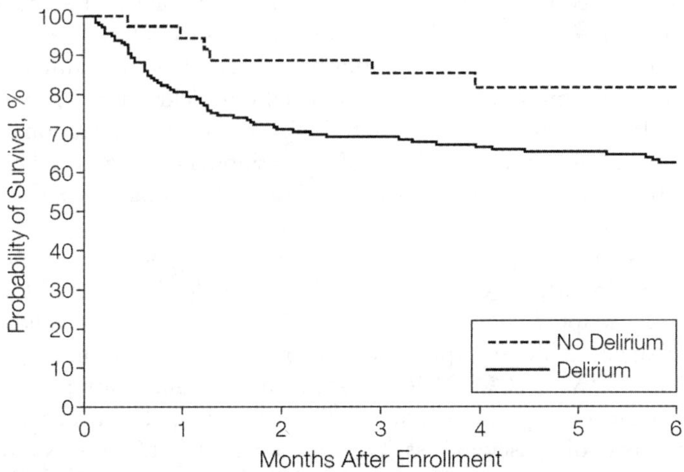

Fig. 1. Delirium in the ICU is associated with a decreased survival rate. (*From* Ely EW, Shintani A, Truman B, et al. Delirium as a predictor of mortality in mechanically ventilated patients in the intensive care unit. JAMA 2004;291(14):1753–62; with permission.)

complications, be discharged to a rehabilitation facility, develop posttraumatic stress disorder, and develop long-term cognitive dysfunction [17–19].

HYPOACTIVE, HYPERACTIVE, AND MIXED TYPES OF DELIRIUM

There are three subtypes of delirium: hyperactive, hypoactive, and mixed forms.

Hyperactive delirium is the form most obvious to the clinician and is characterized by restless and unusual behavior that often leads to disruptions in patient care. Although this agitated behavior pattern may be the behavior pattern most associated with delirium, pure hyperactive delirium is the least common form [20,21].

Hypoactive delirium is characterized by lethargy, inattentiveness, and the signs and symptoms of depression. The negative symptoms of hypoactive delirium often lead to its misdiagnosis, because these symptoms are mistaken for depression or dementia, or are simply attributed to old age. Although patients with hypoactive delirium are the least likely to disrupt their medical care, diagnosing and treating them is very important because they have the greatest morbidity and mortality of all patients with delirium [22].

The mixed-type delirium involves intermittent symptoms of both the hyperactive and hypoactive forms of delirium. This form of delirium is the most common.

DIAGNOSTIC TOOLS

The symptoms of delirium are numerous, can vary both between patients and within the same patient over time, and are shared by a variety of other disorders, which can often lead to delays in diagnosis and treatment. In one study, nurses and physicians correctly diagnosed delirium in only 28% of patients [23]. Although several quick and easy-to-administer delirium screening tests have been available for several years, the American College of Critical Care Medicine began to recommend routine monitoring for delirium in all ICU patients only after mounting evidence showed that delirium is an independent predictor of morbidity and mortality [24]. A recent multinational survey, however, found that only 33% of ICU practitioners use a specific delirium screening protocol on a routine basis, indicating that much progress can still be made [25].

The most widely used screening tool for identifying delirium at the bedside has been the Confusion Assessment Method (CAM). The related CAM-ICU protocol was adapted for use in nonverbal patients and was validated in 2 major investigations for its specificity and reliability in determining delirium [10,26]. The CAM and CAM-ICU assess the 4 main features of delirium, including acute change in mental status, inattention, disorganized thinking, and altered level of consciousness (Fig. 2); the CAM-ICU assesses the absence or presence of these features. The test is easily administered by a trained ICU nurse and has high positive and negative predictive value in this setting. A recent study indicates that the CAM-ICU may be the best bedside diagnostic tool currently available [27].

A

Scale	Label	Description
+4	COMBATIVE	Combative, violent, immediate danger to staff
+3	VERY AGITATED	Pulls to remove tubes or catheters; aggressive
+2	AGITATED	Frequent non-purposeful movement, fights ventilator
+1	RESTLESS	Anxious, apprehensive, movements not aggressive
0	ALERT & CALM	Spontaneously pays attention to caregiver
-1	DROWSY	Not fully alert, but has sustained awakening to voice (eye opening & contact >10 sec)
-2	LIGHT SEDATION	Briefly awakens to voice (eyes open & contact <10 sec)
-3	MODERATE SEDATION	Movement or eye opening to voice (no eye contact)
-4	DEEP SEDATION	No response to voice, but movement or eye opening to physical stimulation
-5	UNAROUSEABLE	No response to voice or physical stimulation

B

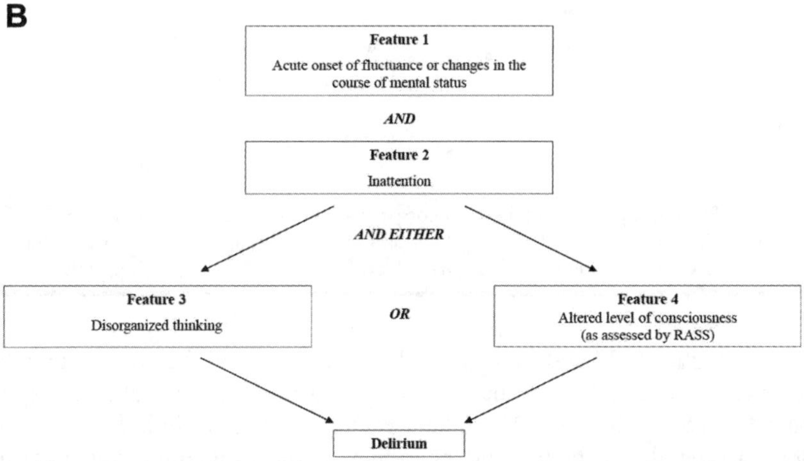

Fig. 2. CAM-ICU. (*A*) Step 1: assess level of sedation with the Richmond Agitation-Sedation Scale. (*B*) Step 2: assess for the presence of delirium with the CAM-ICU. (*Data from* Sessler CN, Gosnell M, Grap MJ, et al. The Richmond Agitation-Sedation Scale: validity and reliability in adult intensive care patients. Am J Respir Crit Care Med 2002;166:1338–44 and Ely EW, Margolin R, Francis J, et al. Evaluation of delirium in critically ill patients: validation of the Confusion Assessment Method for the Intensive Care Unit (CAM-ICU). Crit Care Med 2001;29(7):1370–9.)

DELIRIUM INCREASES THE COST OF MEDICAL CARE

The cost impact of delirium is substantial. A study of 500 patients undergoing elective surgery found an 11.4% delirium rate associated with a 23% increased length of stay, leading to an 18% increase in nursing costs ($5,333 vs $4,353) and a 22% increase in total cost ($11,762 vs $9,145). These numbers did not include the additional costs of postacute care (eg, nursing home placement, home health) [28]. Another study examined the costs associated with delirium in the mechanically ventilated patient. After adjustment for age, comorbidity, severity of illness, and other potential confounders, delirium was associated

A

	Non Delirium Group	Delirium Group
Adjusted total cost per day survived	$166	$461
Adjusted total annual health care cost	$49,452-59,833	$65,755-120,349

B

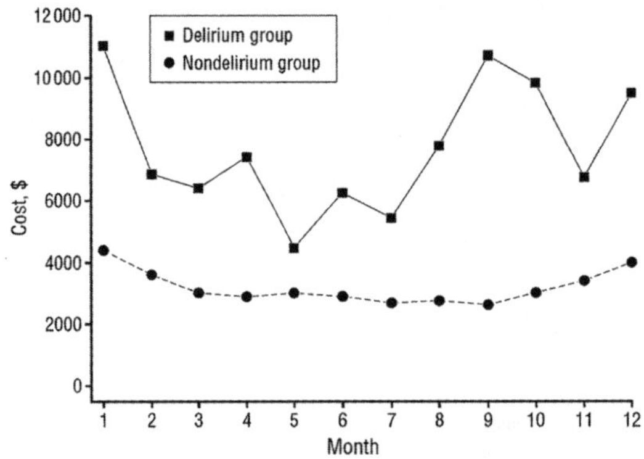

Fig. 3. (*A, B*) Adjusted mean total health care costs are increased in patients with delirium. (*From* Leslie DL, Marcantonio ER, Zhang Y, et al. One-year health care costs associated with delirium in the elderly population. Arch Intern Med 2008;168:27–32; with permission.)

with 39% higher ICU and 31% higher hospital costs [29]. Further cost analysis studies estimate that the national burden of delirium on the health care system ranges from $38 billion to $152 billion each year (Fig. 3) [30]. Therefore, it is not surprising that a better understanding of the prevention and treatment options of delirium has become a major public health care goal.

PATHOPHYSIOLOGY

The pathophysiology of delirium is poorly understood but is likely multifactorial. Decreased oxygen carrying capacity is implicated in the development of delirium. In one study, postthoracotomy patients with low arterial oxygen saturation had an increased risk of developing delirium. In all patients who developed delirium in this study, supplemental oxygen raised arterial oxygen saturation and resolved their delirium, indicating that hypoxemia may contribute to postoperative delirium [31].

Research has emphasized the potential importance of systemic inflammation as an underlying mechanism for delirium. The systemic inflammation leads to tissue damage causing breakdown of the blood-brain barrier and changes in the neuronal signaling [32]. Indeed, patients undergoing surgery for hip fractures were found to have higher levels of C-reactive protein which is released in response to acute inflammation. This finding supports the hypothesis that inflammation may lead to brain injury and subsequently to delirium [33, 34].

Dysregulation of several neurotransmitters, including acetylcholine, gamma-aminobutyric acid (GABA), dopamine, and serotonin, has been implicated in the development of delirium. Drugs with anticholinergic properties, including atropine, meperidine, diphenhydramine, and tricyclic antidepressants, are known to directly contribute to delirium. The protective role of acetylcholine against the development of a neuroinflammatory response is supported by the finding that it activates pathways which block the synthesis of proinflammatory cytokines [35].

Benzodiazepines and other sedatives and hypnotics (including alcohol, barbiturates, and propofol) act, at least partly, via GABA-receptor stimulation. The mechanism through which these medications induce delirium is again multifactorial, but is thought to include disturbance in the normal sleep/wake pattern. Perturbations in GABA signaling are also implicated in hepatic encephalopathy, a form of altered cognition that is in many ways similar to delirium. In one double-blind, placebo-controlled study, the benzodiazepine antagonist flumazenil was found to have a beneficial effect on acute hepatic encephalopathy [36].

Dopamine, which tends to have excitatory effects, has been implicated as a risk factor for delirium when given exogenously, and endogenous dopaminergic hyperfunction via upregulated dopamine receptors is thought to contribute to the development of delirium [37].

PREVENTION AND THE ROLE OF THE ANESTHESIOLOGIST

Because of the multifactorial origin of delirium, a multicomponent strategy aimed at preventing delirium seems most promising. In a landmark trial, Inouye and colleagues [38] evaluated 852 hospitalized patients who were randomly assigned to usual care or management with a multicomponent intervention, including a nonpharmacologic sleep protocol, early mobilization activities, range of motion exercises, timely removal of catheters and physical restraints, use of eyeglasses and hearing aids, and early correction of dehydration. These interventions significantly reduced the incidence of delirium (15% in the usual care group vs 9.9% in the intervention group).

Although patient, surgical, and postoperative care factors are likely more important to the development of delirium than the choice of anesthesia, anesthesiologists can reduce the risk of developing postoperative delirium in several notable ways. First, anesthesiologists can identify patients at increased risk for developing delirium during the preoperative evaluation through assessing the patient's physical and mental status and their medications. In older patients with multiple risk factors for delirium, the mainstays of good intraoperative care must be continued, such as maintaining normal oxygenation, blood pressure, and electrolyte levels.

Several studies and a recent meta-analysis have shown no difference in the incidence of postoperative delirium during either general or regional anesthesia [39]. A recent small randomized controlled trial, however, indicated that the level of sedation during regional anesthesia is an important risk factor for the development of postoperative delirium. In this study, patients undergoing hip surgery with spinal anesthesia were randomized to either a deep sedation group, in which the average bispectral index (BIS) was approximately 50, or a light sedation group with a BIS of 80 or greater. The incidence of delirium was 41% in the deep sedation group, and only 19% in the light sedation cohort [40]. These data are intriguing because they suggest that a delirium-causing component of regional anesthesia may be the "deep" sedation that often accompanies it. Although further studies are necessary to test this hypothesis directly, these data support the theory that less sedation is better in patients with multiple risk factors for delirium.

PHARMACOLOGIC APPROACH TO DELIRIUM REDUCTION

Medications are often the precipitating factor for episodes of delirium. The medications routinely administered in the perioperative period are also known to be some of the worst offenders, including benzodiazepines, opioids, corticosteroids, and medications with significant anticholinergic activity. Although the use of many of these medications is often necessary, the goal is to reduce their use to dosages required for medical effect. In general, drugs with short elimination half-lives are preferable to long-acting drugs. The authors suggest to incorporate the following considerations into the anesthetic plan.

1. Benzodiazepines: the amount of benzodiazepines given is directly related to the incidence and severity of delirium [7]. The anesthesiologist should carefully weigh the benefit of administering benzodiazepines against the potential risk for delirium, and consider abstaining from their use in patients with multiple risk factors for delirium.
2. Opioids: although many studies have indicated that opioids contribute to or cause delirium, increased postoperative pain is also directly correlated with an increased risk of delirium [41]. Anesthesia providers must strike a delicate balance between adequate pain control and avoiding overmedication.
3. Anticholinergic medications: atropine and scopolamine should be used only if necessary, because a decrease in acetylcholine activity in the brain is implicated in the development of delirium. Glycopyrrolate may be a better choice than atropine, because it is a quaternary amine and has less blood-brain barrier penetration than atropine. Other medications with anticholinergic properties, including diphenhydramine and tricyclic antidepressants, are also well-known to increase the risk of delirium [42,43].
4. When choosing an inotrope, dopamine should be avoided because increased dopamine activity has been implicated in the development of delirium [37].
5. Emerging data show a benefit to the use of dexmedetomidine for sedation over other sedatives. One recent study showed that intubated ICU patients receiving dexmedetomidine were mechanically ventilated for shorter times, experienced less delirium, and developed less tachycardia and hypertension [44]. Moreover, a recent small study comparing mortality in septic patients receiving either dexmedetomidine or lorazepam showed a reduced mortality rate in the dexmedetomidine group [45]. These findings are intriguing, because dexmedetomidine, an α-agonist, is thought to spare the GABA-receptor pathway, and may potentiate endogenous sleep-promoting pathways.

6. Early extubation should be a high priority. Receiving fewer and less sedatives while intubated may reduce the chance of developing delirium, and therefore decrease morbidity and mortality.
7. Acetylcholinesterase inhibitors, which have been useful in the treatment of symptoms associated with Alzheimer disease, have not been shown to decrease the risk of postoperative delirium. In fact, a double-blind, randomized, controlled trial of rivastigmine for the treatment of ICU delirium had to be stopped early because of an increased mortality in the treatment group. Although no significant difference in delirium symptoms was seen between the study groups, the rivastigmine treatment group showed a trend toward longer delirium duration [46]. Given the increased mortality associated with its use and the lack of benefit in delirium treatment, the use of rivastigmine in the treatment of delirium in the ICU is not recommended.

TREATMENT

The U.S. Food and Drug Administration has not currently approved any medication for the treatment of delirium. Although the first goal in treating delirium is to identify and treat any underlying medical conditions that may be causing or contributing to delirium, if medication is to be used, choices include first-generation antipsychotics (haloperidol) and second-generation (atypical) antipsychotics (eg, olanzapine and risperidone). Although second-generation antipsychotics may have a decreased incidence of side effects, there is less published experience using these medications in hospitalized patients for the treatment of delirium than with haloperidol.

Several attempts have been made to reduce the incidence of postoperative delirium through prophylactic medical treatment. Haloperidol was evaluated as a prophylactic therapy for the prevention of postoperative delirium in elderly patients undergoing hip surgery. Kalisvaart conducted a randomized, double-blind, placebo-controlled trial in 430 elderly hip surgery patients and found that 1.5 mg/d of haloperidol significantly reduced the severity and duration of delirium [47]. Others, however, have urged caution in interpreting these findings, because a reduction in the severity of delirium symptoms could be explained by a conversion from the hyperactive form of delirium to the more morbid hypoactive form [6,48].

POSTOPERATIVE DELIRIUM AND POSTOPERATIVE COGNITIVE DYSFUNCTION

The differential diagnosis of delirium includes postoperative cognitive dysfunction (POCD). POCD is a deterioration of cognition that occurs weeks to months after surgery and anesthesia. This time frame is one of the principal distinctions between POCD and postoperative delirium; postoperative delirium occurs hours to days (typically 24–72 hours) after surgery, whereas POCD is measured at weeks to months after surgery and anesthesia (Table 1) [49]. POCD is a persistent change in cognitive performance for at least several months, whereas delirium tends to be transient. Because of the wide variability in normal human cognitive capacities, baseline measurements of cognitive

Table 1
Distinction between postoperative delirium and postoperative cognitive dysfunction

Postoperative delirium	POCD
• Change in mental status o Reduced level of consciousness • Acute onset typically 1–3 d after surgery • Fluctuating symptoms • Duration of days to weeks • Reversible	• Deterioration in cognition o Normal level of consciousness • Pernicious onset after surgery • Persistent symptoms • Duration of weeks to months or longer • Often reversible

function before surgery/anesthesia are a critical component when evaluating patients for POCD. In the absence of baseline data, low postoperative test scores cannot be associated with surgical, anesthetic, or illness variables with any certainty.

Despite the distinguishing characteristics of postoperative delirium and POCD, there is likely a continuum between the two syndromes. Levkoff and colleagues [50] found that only 21% of patients with delirium returned to their baseline cognitive function 3 months after discharge, and only 49% at 6 months. Another study found a significant association between the duration of delirium and short-term POCD, suggesting that attention deficits may place delirium and POCD on a continuum of the postoperatively disordered brain [51]. In the future, studies that undertake sophisticated evaluations for both postoperative delirium and POCD should improve understanding of this issue.

SUMMARY

Postoperative delirium is a change in cognition in the postoperative period that occurs frequently, particularly in the elderly. It is a major public health concern that negatively affects morbidity and mortality and places a large fiscal burden on the health care system. Although anesthesiologists' care often ends well before symptoms of postoperative delirium begin, they can play an important role in the prevention of this disease.

References

[1] American Psychiatric Association. Diagnostic and statistical manual of mental disorder: fourth edition DSM-IV-TR. Arlington, Virginia: Amer Psychiatric Pub; 2000.

[2] Gustafson Y, Berggren D, Brännström B, et al. Acute confusional states in elderly patients treated for femoral neck fracture. J Am Geriatr Soc 1988;36(6):525–30.

[3] Dyer CB, Ashton CM, Teasdale TA. Postoperative delirium: a review of 80 primary data-collection studies. Arch Intern Med 1995;155(5):461–5.

[4] Maldonado JR. Delirium in the acute care setting: characteristics, diagnosis and treatment. Crit Care Clin 2008;24(4):657–722, vii.

[5] Maldonado JR. Pathoetiological model of delirium: a comprehensive understanding of the neurobiology of delirium and an evidence-based approach to prevention and treatment. Crit Care Clin 2008;24(4):789–856, ix.

[6] Rudolph JL, Marcantonio ER. Postoperative delirium: acute change with long-term implications. Anesth Analg 2011;112(5):1202–11.

[7] Pandharipande P, Shintani A, Peterson J, et al. Lorazepam is an independent risk factor for transitioning to delirium in intensive care unit patients. Anesthesiology 2006;104(1):21–6.
[8] Lowery DP, Wesnes K, Ballard CG. Subtle attentional deficits in the absence of dementia are associated with an increased risk of post-operative delirium. Dement Geriatr Cogn Disord 2007;23(6):390–4.
[9] McNicoll L, Pisani MA, Zhang Y, et al. Delirium in the intensive care unit: occurrence and clinical course in older patients. J Am Geriatr Soc 2003;51(5):591–8.
[10] Ely EW, Inouye SK, Bernard GR, et al. Delirium in mechanically ventilated patients validity and reliability of the Confusion Assessment Method for the Intensive Care Unit (CAM-ICU). JAMA 2001;286(21):2703–10.
[11] Peterson JF, Pun BT, Dittus RS, et al. Delirium and its motoric subtypes: a study of 614 critically ill patients. J Am Geriatr Soc 2006;54(3):479–84.
[12] Aldemir M, Özen S, Kara IH, et al. Predisposing factors for delirium in the surgical intensive care unit. Crit Care 2001;5(5):265.
[13] Girard TD, Pandharipande PP, Ely EW. Delirium in the intensive care unit. Crit Care 2008;12(Suppl 3):S3.
[14] Fong HK, Sands LP, Leung JM. The role of postoperative analgesia in delirium and cognitive decline in elderly patients: a systematic review. Anesth Analg 2006;102(4):1255–66.
[15] Ely EW, Gautam S, Margolin R, et al. The impact of delirium in the intensive care unit on hospital length of stay. Intensive Care Med 2001;27(12):1892–900.
[16] Kiely DK, Marcantonio ER, Inouye SK, et al. Persistent delirium predicts greater mortality. J Am Geriatr Soc 2009;57(1):55–61.
[17] Francis J, Martin D, Kapoor WN. A prospective study of delirium in hospitalized elderly. JAMA 1990;263(8):1097–101.
[18] Jones C, Griffiths RD, Humphris G, et al. Memory, delusions, and the development of acute posttraumatic stress disorder-related symptoms after intensive care. Crit Care Med 2001;29(3):573–80.
[19] Griffiths RD, Jones C. Delirium, cognitive dysfunction and posttraumatic stress disorder. Curr Opin Anaesthesiol 2007;20(2):124–9.
[20] Meagher DJ, O'Hanlon D, O'Mahony E, et al. Relationship between symptoms and motoric subtype of delirium. J Neuropsychiatry Clin Neurosci 2000;12(1):51–6.
[21] Robinson TN, Raeburn CD, Tran ZV, et al. Motor subtypes of postoperative delirium in older adults. Arch Surg 2011;146(3):295–300.
[22] Kiely DK, Jones RN, Bergmann MA, et al. Association between psychomotor activity delirium subtypes and mortality among newly admitted postacute facility patients. J Gerontol A Biol Sci Med Sci 2007;62(2):174–9.
[23] Collins N, Blanchard MR, Tookman A, et al. Detection of delirium in the acute hospital. Age Ageing 2010;39(1):131–5.
[24] Jacobi J, Fraser GL, Coursin DB, et al. Clinical practice guidelines for the sustained use of sedatives and analgesics in the critically ill adult. Crit Care Med 2002;30(1):119–41.
[25] Patel RP, Gambrell M, Speroff T, et al. Delirium and sedation in the intensive care unit: survey of behaviors and attitudes of 1384 healthcare professionals. Crit Care Med 2009;37(3):825–32.
[26] Ely EW, Margolin R, Francis J, et al. Evaluation of delirium in critically ill patients: validation of the Confusion Assessment Method for the Intensive Care Unit (CAM-ICU). Crit Care Med 2001;29(7):1370–9.
[27] Wong CL, Holroyd-Leduc J, Simel DL, et al. Does this patient have delirium?: value of bedside instruments. JAMA 2010;304(7):779–86.
[28] Franco K, Litaker D, Locala J, et al. The cost of delirium in the surgical patient. Psychosomatics 2001;42(1):68–73.
[29] Milbrandt EB, Deppen S, Harrison PL, et al. Costs associated with delirium in mechanically ventilated patients. Crit Care Med 2004;32(4):955–62.

[30] Leslie DL, Marcantonio ER, Zhang Y, et al. One-year health care costs associated with delirium in the elderly population. Arch Intern Med 2008;168(1):27–32.
[31] Aakerlund LP, Rosenberg J. Postoperative delirium: treatment with supplementary oxygen. Br J Anaesth 1994;72(3):286–90.
[32] Meyer NJ, Hall JB. Brain dysfunction in critically ill patients–the intensive care unit and beyond. Crit Care 2006;10(4):223.
[33] Beloosesky Y, Hendel D, Weiss A, et al. Cytokines and C-reactive protein production in hip-fracture-operated elderly patients. J Gerontol A Biol Sci Med Sci 2007;62(4):420–6.
[34] Lee HJ, Hwang DS, Wang SK, et al. Early assessment of delirium in elderly patients after hip surgery. Psychiatry Investig 2011;8(4):340–7.
[35] Czura CJ, Friedman SG, Tracey KJ. Neural inhibition of inflammation: the cholinergic anti-inflammatory pathway. J Endotoxin Res 2003;9(6):409–13.
[36] Laccetti M, Manes G, Uomo G, et al. Flumazenil in the treatment of acute hepatic encephalopathy in cirrhotic patients: a double blind randomized placebo controlled study. Dig Liver Dis 2000;32(4):335–8.
[37] Sommer BR, Wise LC, Kraemer HC. Is dopamine administration possibly a risk factor for delirium? Crit Care Med 2002;30(7):1508–11.
[38] Inouye SK, Bogardus ST Jr, Charpentier PA, et al. A multicomponent intervention to prevent delirium in hospitalized older patients. N Engl J Med 1999;340(9):669–76.
[39] Bryson GL, Wyand A. Evidence-based clinical update: general anesthesia and the risk of delirium and postoperative cognitive dysfunction. Can J Anaesth 2006;53(7):669–77.
[40] Sieber FE, Zakriya KJ, Gottschalk A, et al. Sedation depth during spinal anesthesia and the development of postoperative delirium in elderly patients undergoing hip fracture repair. Mayo Clin Proc 2010;85(1):18–26.
[41] Vaurio LE, Sands LP, Wang Y, et al. Postoperative delirium: the importance of pain and pain management. Anesth Analg 2006;102(4):1267–73.
[42] Oxman TE. Antidepressants and cognitive impairment in the elderly. J Clin Psychiatry 1996;57(Suppl 5):38–44.
[43] Agostini JV, Leo-Summers LS, Inouye SK. Cognitive and other adverse effects of diphenhydramine use in hospitalized older patients. Arch Intern Med 2001;161(17):2091–7.
[44] Riker RR, Shehabi Y, Bokesch PM, et al. Dexmedetomidine vs midazolam for sedation of critically ill patients: a randomized trial. JAMA 2009;301(5):489–99.
[45] Pandharipande PP, Sanders RD, Girard TD, et al. Effect of dexmedetomidine versus lorazepam on outcome in patients with sepsis: an a priori-designed analysis of the MENDS randomized controlled trial. Crit Care 2010;14(2):R38.
[46] van Eijk MM, Roes KC, Honing ML, et al. Effect of rivastigmine as an adjunct to usual care with haloperidol on duration of delirium and mortality in critically ill patients: a multicentre, double-blind, placebo-controlled randomised trial. Lancet 2010;376(9755):1829–37.
[47] Kalisvaart KJ, de Jonghe JF, Bogaards MJ, et al. Haloperidol prophylaxis for elderly hip-surgery patients at risk for delirium: a randomized placebo-controlled study. J Am Geriatr Soc 2005;53(10):1658–66.
[48] Marcantonio ER, Bergmann MA, Kiely DK, et al. Response letter to Dr. Pitkälä and colleagues. J Am Geriatr Soc 2011;59(1):168–9.
[49] Silverstein JH, Timberger M, Reich DL, et al. Central nervous system dysfunction after noncardiac surgery and anesthesia in the elderly. Anesthesiology 2007;106(3):622–8.
[50] Levkoff SE, Evans DA, Liptzin B, et al. Delirium. The occurrence and persistence of symptoms among elderly hospitalized patients. Arch Intern Med 1992;152(2):334–40.
[51] Rudolph JL, Marcantonio ER, Culley DJ, et al. Delirium is associated with early postoperative cognitive dysfunction. Anaesthesia 2008;63(9):941–7.

Advances in Anesthesia 30 (2012) 13–27

ADVANCES IN ANESTHESIA

ELSEVIER
MOSBY

Consciousness and Anesthesia

An Update for the Clinician

Magnus K. Teig, MBChB, MRCP, FRCA[a],
Anthony G. Hudetz, DBM, PhD[b,c,d],
George A. Mashour, MD, PhD[a,*]

[a]Department of Anesthesiology, University of Michigan Medical School, 1500 East Medical Center Drive, UH 1H247, Ann Arbor, MI 48109-5048, USA; [b]Department of Anesthesiology, Medical College of Wisconsin, 8701 Watertown Plank Road, Milwaukee, WI 53226, USA; [c]Department of Physiology, Medical College of Wisconsin, 8701 Watertown Plank Road, Milwaukee, WI 53226, USA; [d]Department of Biophysics, Medical College of Wisconsin, 8701 Watertown Plank Road, Milwaukee, WI 53226, USA

Keywords
• Consciousness • Anesthesia • Intraoperative awareness • Brain monitoring

Key Points

- Intraoperative awareness with explicit recall occurs in 1 to 2 cases per thousand and is linked to the neuroscientific problem of consciousness.
- Current brain monitoring techniques may be useful in preventing awareness during routine care or total intravenous anesthesia (TIVA) but are not superior to protocols based on anesthetic concentration.
- Real-time measure of functional and directional connectivity across different brain regions known to be important for consciousness may be the next wave of intraoperative brain monitors.

INTRODUCTION

It is 7:18 AM on a Tuesday morning and you are standing in the preoperative holding area. In front of you is the first patient of the day, a normally self-assured individual looking decidedly nervous. After the history and physical

Funding sources: Dr Teig–none; Dr Hudetz is supported by the National Institutes of Health, RO1GM56398; Dr Mashour is supported by National Institutes of Health, RO1GM098578.

Conflict of interest: Dr Teig–none; Dr Hudetz–none; Dr Mashour–holds a provisional patent on the use of directional connectivity for brain monitoring.

*Corresponding author. Department of Anesthesiology, University of Michigan Medical School, 1500 East Medical Center Drive, UH 1H247, Ann Arbor, MI 48109-5048. *E-mail address*: gmashour@umich.edu

0737-6146/12/$ – see front matter
http://dx.doi.org/10.1016/j.aan.2012.08.001

examination are complete, she looks at you intently and asks, "How will you *know* that I am unconscious during my surgery?"

First reported in 1846 in the original description of etherization by Bigelow [1], the history of intraoperative awareness is as old as the field of anesthesiology itself. In the most extreme cases, a patient may be able to describe in vivid and horrifying detail every event, conversation, and sensation that occurred during a painful operation (see Rowan [2] for a first-person description from a physician). The unintended experience of intraoperative events can have potentially catastrophic psychological consequences, with a high proportion of patients developing posttraumatic stress disorder [3].

This clinical update on consciousness and memory formation during surgery reviews the clinical definition, epidemiology, risk factors, and prevention of intraoperative awareness with explicit recall as well as new directions in the monitoring of anesthetic-induced unconsciousness.

DEFINITION OF AWARENESS

In the cognitive sciences, *awareness* denotes subjective experience alone, but in clinical anesthesiology it has become shorthand for multiple cognitive processes:

Awareness = consciousness + recall

Recall may be classified as explicit (a form of conscious memory) or implicit (a form of unconscious memory). Studies addressing awareness are concerned with explicit episodic memory. Awareness during surgery may thus be more accurately regarded as the failure to suppress consciousness (comprised of arousal and experience) and the ability to form explicit episodic memories of intraoperative events [4]. To date there is no objective way for the assessment of subjective experience in a paralyzed or otherwise noncommunicating patient [5].

Consciousness is possibly the greatest unanswered question in science. Its enigma has dominated the thinking of some of the greatest scientific minds throughout history, from Socrates and Plato in the fifth century BC to Nobel Prize–winning scientists of the modern era, such as Francis Crick [6] and Gerald Edelman [7]. The term, *consciousness*, can be further subdivided as connected consciousness and disconnected consciousness [8]. Connected consciousness refers to consciousness of external or environmental stimuli, whereas disconnected consciousness refers to internally conscious states, such as dreaming, in which an individual is unresponsive to environmental input. Both of these forms of consciousness are dissociable from explicit episodic recall (ie, individuals may be conscious of external or internal events without remembering them).

An example of this phenomenon is that responsiveness to commands under anesthesia, demonstrated by the isolated forearm technique, is often not associated with memory. In a recent review [8], 37% of patients assessed with the isolated forearm technique could follow auditory commands and thus had connected consciousness, but only 25% of those who responded under anesthesia had any recall of events. These patients were connected with their environment but lack the ability to form memories and thus could not be said to suffer from awareness as clinically defined in anesthesiology. It is highly likely that far more patients experience intraoperative consciousness than awareness with explicit recall. Disconnected consciousness, even with associated explicit recall of dream content, is also considered distinct from what is conventionally defined as awareness. For example, dreaming under anesthesia with explicit recall is common and may occur in approximately 1 in 4 patients [9]. It is now clear that dreams during anesthesia are not necessarily near-miss awareness events.

EPIDEMIOLOGY OF AWARENESS

Incidence of awareness

Awareness has been consistently reported across several large studies, using the modified Brice interview [10], as occurring in 1/1000 to 2/1000 of anesthetics, with some recent studies reporting an incidence of up to 1%. Discrepancies in rate of incidence may relate to the definition of awareness used (Table 1).

Describing the severity of awareness

Classification tools have been developed to assess the qualitative aspects of the awareness experience. The Michigan Awareness Classification Instrument [15] is one such classification (Box 1).

The Michigan Awareness Classification Instrument has good interobserver reliability, allows for statistical analysis of the severity of awareness, and may help the study of interventions to reduce awareness and postawareness sequelae.

RISK FACTORS FOR AWARENESS

Because intraoperative awareness is a rare event, our understanding of the risk factors is imprecise. Observational studies over decades have attempted to characterize risk factors for awareness [16]. Over time, however, there have been substantial changes in clinical practice, so it may be the case that both the incidence and risk factors for awareness have changed accordingly [4].

Two broad groups of patients are most at risk for awareness:

1. Those who receive an insufficient dose of anesthetic drug from their anesthesia provider

Table 1
Major studies of awareness incidence

Study, year	Population—location	Incidence	Percent aware
Sandin et al [11], 2000	Adult—Sweden	19/11,785	0.16
Sebel et al [12], 2004	Adult—US	25/19.575	0.13
Errando et al [13], 2008	Adult—Spain	39/3921	1.0
Davidson et al [14], 2011	Pediatric—multiple	33/4486	0.73

Box 1: Michigan Awareness Classification Instrument

Class 0: no awareness

Class 1: isolated auditory perceptions

Class 2: tactile perceptions (eg, surgical manipulation of endotracheal tube)

Class 3: pain

Class 4: paralysis (eg, feeling one cannot move, speak, or breathe)

Class 5: paralysis and pain

An additional designation of *D* for distress is included for patient reports of fear, anxiety, suffocation, sense of doom, sense of impending death, and so forth. If multiple experiences are reported, the highest classification category is used.

2. Those who receive what is typically considered a sufficient dose but are resistant to anesthetic effects

Underdosed patients

Anesthesia providers may chose deliberately to give a patient a minimal dose of anesthetic drug because of physiologic instability or to prevent physiologic instability in a fetus [16–19]. There are also situations, however, in which anesthesia providers unintentionally deliver inadequate anesthesia, such as with vaporizer failure, interrupted intravenous anesthesia, or during difficult intubations in which there is no redosing of a sedative-hypnotic.

Patient resistance factors

Patients may have an acquired or intrinsic resistance to the anesthetic effects. Patients who may have an acquired resistance to anesthetic drugs include

1. Regular users of benzodiazepines, opiates, or other drugs that affect the cytochrome P450 enzyme system, such as alcohol
2. Regular users of other upregulators of the cytochrome P450 3A enzyme pathway (ie, St. John's wort, efavirenz, nevirapine, barbiturates, carbamazepine, glucocorticoids, phenytoin, and rifampin) [20], who conceivably might also have increase resistance to anesthesia

Certain genetic mutations, notably the melanocortin 1 receptor gene mutation, which confers red hair phenotype, may cause increased resistance to inhalation anesthesia [21]. Another example of a genetic contribution to anesthetic sensitivity is resistance to the amnesic effects of etomidate [22] or isoflurane [23] conferred by the presence of an $\alpha5$ subunit mutation of the $GABA_A$ receptor. It is possible that other, as yet unknown, genetic mutations may also be linked with anesthesia resistance or susceptibility.

Patients at high risk of awareness have been grouped together for study in multicenter trials of awareness, aiming to increase the power of these studies. The risk factors used in the largest study of awareness to date, the BIS or Anesthesia Gas to Reduce Explicit Recall trial [24], are listed in Box 2.

Box 2: Risk Factors for Intraoperative Awareness

Planned open heart surgery
Aortic stenosis
Pulmonary hypertension
Use of opiates
Use of benzodiazepines
Use of anticonvulsant drugs
Daily alcohol consumption
American Society of Anesthesiologists status 4
End-stage lung disease
History of intraoperative awareness
History of or anticipated difficult intubation
Cardiac ejection fraction <40%
Marginal exercise tolerance

Note that emergency or obstetric cases were not included in this study but are also risk factors.

Data from Avidan MS, Jacobsohn E, Glick D, et al. Prevention of intraoperative awareness in a high-risk surgical population. N Engl J Med 2011;365:591–600.

What can be done to prevent awareness? As with all aspects of anesthesia practice, attention to detail is the key; a checklist-based approach minimize the chance of awareness (Box 3).

Muscle relaxants compound the risk of anesthetic underdosing by preventing patients' ability to signal distress. In one study, the incidence of awareness was 0.18% when muscle relaxants were used versus 0.10% without [11]. In another, all patients who reported awareness had received muscle relaxants, reporting the inability to move as the most distressing sensation [13].

Anesthetic technique used, as well as type and timing of surgery, has been implicated in increasing the frequency of awareness. TIVA is associated with a higher frequency of awareness [25] versus inhalational agents. This may be because there is currently no standard dosing metric for TIVA that can be monitored intraoperatively, so anesthetic delivery failure might be missed.

MEASURING THE DEPTH OF ANESTHESIA

Depth of anesthesia was initially described as a classification of clinical observations in response to a single inhaled agent, ether. First described by John Snow in 1847 [26] and formalized in 1937 by Guedel [27], these "planes" are now rarely seen in the modern era of rapid induction with intravenous drugs.

Modern measures of anesthesia depth rely on either 1 or both of 2 modalities:

1. End-tidal drug monitoring
2. EEG-based techniques

Box 3: Awareness prevention checklist

- Equipment and drug check, including dosages: Are all drugs labeled and infusions running into veins?
- Consider an amnesic premedication or redosing in patients at high risk, such as those with a history of awareness.
- Avoid muscle relaxants or minimize the dose given with nerve stimulator monitoring.
- Use a potent inhalational agent rather than total intravenous anesthesia, if possible.
- Set a minimum alveolar concentration (MAC) alarm to at least 0.5 to 0.7.
- If on cardiac bypass, monitor anesthetic agent concentration within the circuit.
- Treat hypotension by means other than reducing the anesthetic concentration.
- If concerned about hemodynamic compromise, use drugs with the widest therapeutic index; administer benzodiazepines or scopolamine.
- Supplement hypnotic agents with systemic opioid or local analgesia to minimize experience of pain if awareness occurs.
- Consider use of a brain monitor (ie, raw or processed electroencephalogram [EEG]).
- Routinely monitor the brain if using total intravenous anesthesia.
- Evaluate known risk factors for awareness; consider if a higher dose of anesthetic may be required.
- Redose the intravenous anesthetic if intubation is difficult or prolonged or during rigid bronchoscopy.

Modified from Mashour GA, Orser BA, Avidan MS. Intraoperative awareness: from neurobiology to clinical practice. Anesthesiology 2011;114:1218–33.

Minimum alveolar concentration–based techniques

Calculation of the MAC, which reflects a common expression of anesthetic dosing, dates from 1965 [28]. Pharmacologically, MAC is the ED_{50} (ie, the effective dose at which 50% of the population does not move in response to a standard noxious stimulus). The concept of MAC has since been expanded to include MAC-awake, the MAC at which 50% of the population regains consciousness, which is usually noted at between 0.3 to 0.5 MAC.

MAC alarms have been demonstrated to reduce the risk of awareness. An awareness rate of 2/2852 (0.07%) of patients in a surgical population deemed at high risk of awareness (in which the expected incidence is up to 1%) was achieved using alarms set to 0.7 MAC [24]. MAC is a reliable metric but is limited to inhaled anesthetics, motivating the use of end-organ monitors, such as the EEG.

EEG-based techniques

EEG-based anesthesia monitoring technologies fall into 2 general categories: spontaneous EEG (raw or processed) and evoked potentials. There is an extensive range of monitors available, reviewed elsewhere [29]. Clinical anesthesiologists can be trained to interpret a raw EEG at a basic level [30] and even to predict bispectral index (BIS) values with accuracy similar to a second BIS monitor used in tandem [31]. Processed EEG, however, potentially aids interpretation for the untrained and can facilitate numeric thresholds for the purpose of subanesthetic alerts.

There has been an expansion of technologies to process and interpret the raw EEG, putatively producing a measure of the depth of anesthesia. At a basic level, these devices apply Fourier transformation to the EEG signal before analyzing each frequency domain of the EEG or spectrum and its contribution to the total signal [32]. Some devices use a proprietary EEG algorithm, calibrated against observed responses to anesthesia, whereas others use publicly available EEG interpretation algorithms of the entropy within the EEG signal [33]. Many commercially available monitors are broadly comparable in reflecting anesthetic dosing [34].

The most widely used device with the largest record of use in randomized controlled trials is the BIS monitor (Covidien, Boulder, Colorado). BIS uses a proprietary EEG algorithm, which generates values from 0 (EEG silence) to 100 (fully awake), with surgical anesthesia defined as a range of 40 to 60. After the first studies in the late 1990s validating the device [35,36], BIS has been investigated as an awareness monitor in a series of large trials [17,19,24].

Studies of the BIS and awareness

The B-Aware trial was the first randomized multicenter trial comparing BIS monitoring with routine care in a population of 2463 patients deemed at high risk for awareness and demonstrated an 80% relative reduction in awareness versus standard care (2 vs 11 cases) [17]. The B-Unaware trial, a further study of 1941 patients similarly deemed at high risk of awareness, failed to demonstrate a difference in outcome between a BIS-guided and end-tidal anesthetic concentration (ETAC)-guided protocol, with each group reporting 2 cases of awareness [19].

BAG-RECALL, the most recent and largest multicenter trial to date, assessed BIS-guided and MAC-guided protocols in 5713 patients at high risk for awareness. The BAG-RECALL trial demonstrated conclusively that a BIS protocol was not superior to an ETAC protocol in preventing awareness [24]; 7 of 2861 patients (0.24%) monitored with BIS experienced definite awareness versus 2 of 2852 (0.07%) of those in whom ETAC alerts were used. It has been suggested by Cochrane meta-analysis [37] that the BIS may prevent awareness compared with routine care, but in patients receiving potent volatile anesthetics an ETAC-guided protocol is a cost-effective alternative. Furthermore, a multicenter trial recently demonstrated that the BIS reduced awareness incidence in patients receiving TIVA compared with standard care (without target-controlled infusion pumps) [25].

Limitations of the BIS

The BIS monitor and similar technologies that also rely on processed EEG have some practical limitations. Anesthetic drugs, such as ketamine [38] and nitrous oxide [39], do not act by potentiating the effects of γ-aminobutyric acid (GABA); they increase EEG frequency, which can cause a paradoxic increase in the BIS value. Nitrous oxide and ketamine may produce unconsciousness via an excitatory pathway, which is not reflected in the BIS and other processed EEG indices. Xenon also produces atypical changes but to a lesser extent, with initially stable processed EEG indices rising after approximately 1 hour of anesthesia time [40].

It is also unclear how well BIS reflects anesthetic dosing over a clinically relevant range of MAC. Analysis of more than 3 million data points, from 1100 patients, of ETAC versus BIS value demonstrated a poor correlation between and a substantial lag in changes in BIS value versus changes in the ETAC [41]. Furthermore, patients may lose consciousness at one BIS value and regain it at another. Similar hysteresis of drug concentration and processed EEG values seems to occur with TIVA [42]. This is not due to time lags of processed EEG [43], however, but likely to the dissociable neurobiology of induction and emergence [44]. Emergence from anesthesia is dependent on the reactivation of the circuits of arousal, which may not be involved in the mechanism of anesthetic induction [45]. This distinct neurobiology may reflect neural inertia [46], the resistance of the brain to undergo transitions between the conscious and unconscious state and vice versa. Neural inertia explains why the current generation of anesthesia monitors does not demonstrate the same values at the point of loss of consciousness and emergence and implies that there should be a small buffer to awareness if the MAC transiently decreases. Certain patients may have reduced neural inertia, leaving them without this buffer zone and allowing for more rapid state transitions from unconsciousness to consciousness.

For an anesthetic monitor to produce a higher fidelity measure of awareness, new techniques rooted in the neurobiology of consciousness are required. Identifying a common neural correlate of both depressive and excitatory anesthetic-induced unconsciousness is the key to developing a superior monitor of awareness [47].

OBJECTIVE MEASURES OF CONNECTED CONSCIOUSNESS AND MEMORY

Can memory be monitored?

From observations of patients with selective neurologic injuries, it is known that the medial temporal lobe plays a critical role in explicit recall; lesions of the hippocampus may prevent the formation of episodic memory [48]. In particular, an oscillatory pattern in the 4 Hz to 12 Hz, or θ range, has been linked to memory processes in both primates and nonprimates [49]. Certain anesthetics have been shown to slow these θ oscillations [50]; the question of whether this slowing is the cause of memory blockade or merely an epiphenomenon remains unanswered. Because of the location of explicit recall centers in the medial temporal lobe (and thus deep to the cortex), memory monitoring at present seems unlikely.

How is consciousness measured?

There is no discreet consciousness center in the brain. There are several wake-promoting and sleep-promoting nuclei, located within the pons, midbrain, hypothalamus, and basal forebrain. These centers regulate sleep and are hypothesized to coordinate in a flip-flop manner to regulate sleep-wake cycles. Brain arousal and sleep-wake cycles, however, are not sufficient for the subjective dimension of consciousness, because patients in vegetative states may have such cycles in the absence of experience [51]. Furthermore, like the structures of the medial temporal lobe mediating explicit recall, subcortical structures mediating arousal are not amenable to real-time monitoring in the operating room. Cortical and thalamocortical activities are believed more closely related to experiential processing and are accessible to study via multiple neuroimaging modalities.

One currently prevailing consciousness hypothesis is that consciousness depends on the integration of information from dynamic interactions across large-scale neural networks in the brain [52,53,54]. Accordingly, general anesthesia might suppress consciousness by either disrupting [55] or unbinding [56] this integrative process. The key to measuring connected consciousness may lie not in measuring the activity of one specific center or region of the brain but instead in tracking the connectivity across neural areas.

Neuroimaging efforts to assess the effect of anesthetics can be divided into 3 basic categories:

1. Assessment of the effects of anesthesia on baseline activity, reflected by cerebral metabolism and cerebral blood flow
2. Responsiveness of neuronal networks to a sensory input or task
3. Functional, directional, or effective connectivity of networks in the brain.

Suppression of metabolic activity

Positron emission tomography (PET) can be used to assess cerebral metabolic rate (CMR). General anesthetics globally reduce CMR and cerebral blood flow, by 30% to 70% at the point of loss of consciousness from propofol infusion [57], with similar results for isoflurane [58] and midazolam [59]. It is unclear if the reduction in CMR or cerebral blood flow is directly responsible for loss of consciousness or a consequence of altered network interactions. Consciousness can coexist with a low CMR state in certain neurologic conditions [60]. Ketamine increases CMR [61]; thus, the excitatory pathway to unconsciousness does not conform to the patterns of primarily inhibitory anesthetics.

Suppression of the thalamus

PET scanning suggests that thalamic suppression is the common site of action for anesthetics [62], a potential mechanism of unconsciousness shared with non–rapid eye movement (REM) sleep and persistent vegetative state [63]. Preliminary electrophysiologic evidence that thalamic suppression follows cortical suppression in time favors an indirect role in anesthetic-induced unconsciousness rather than a causal one [64]. Furthermore, a recent functional MRI study suggested a more profound functional disconnection with the putamen at the point of propofol-induced unconsciousness, with thalamic connectivity well preserved [65].

Metabolic and functional suppression of frontoparietal networks

The frontoparietal network consists of the prefrontal and superior/posterior parietal cortex and is linked to attention, perception, working memory, and consciousness. The frontoparietal network has been shown to be suppressed during anesthesia, non-REM sleep, seizures, and coma [66]; breakdown in frontoparietal connectivity is associated with loss of consciousness [67]. Conversely, return of function in the frontopatietal network is associated with emergence from vegetative state [51].

MRI assessment of functional connectivity during propofol exposure shows suppression of frontoparietal networks with preserved activity in the sensory cortices, suggesting that anesthetic-induced unconsciousness is a higher-order process [68]. Neuroimaging studies also confirm that propofol disrupts functional interactions between sensory and high-order processing systems preventing the conscious perception of incoming stimuli [68]. This breakdown in communication between the higher and lower cortical processing networks seems key in losing consciousness. In support of this, the induction of anesthesia is associated with a loss of effective connectivity (implying causal interactions) across the cortex, as measured by EEG [69].

EEG-based connectivity in frontoparietal networks

Current neuroradiologic techniques have advanced understanding of anesthetic-induced unconsciousness but have poor temporal resolution and are impractical for the operating room. One potential method to assess consciousness is to measure cortical effective connectivity and, in particular, feedback connectivity from the anterior to posterior areas of the brain [70]. For example, evoking activity within the primary visual cortex and its associated feed-forward pathway to higher processing areas is not necessarily associated with conscious experience; a feedback pathway is required [71]. In non-REM sleep and propofol anesthesia, the anterior-to-posterior propagation of slow waves is similar [72,73] and may lead to a disruption of directional connectivity that is common to the 2 states.

EEG studies have demonstrated that frontal-to-parietal feedback connectivity is preferentially inhibited by propofol in healthy volunteers [74] and both propofol and sevoflurane in surgical patients [75]. Feedback connectivity has also been shown to increase during recovery from general anesthesia (Fig. 1) [74–76]; the importance of frontoparietal connectivity in recovery from anesthesia has been confirmed by a recent PET study [77]. Selective disruption of feedback connectivity occurs not only in anesthesia but also in vegetative states, whereas in minimally conscious states directional connectivity patterns are similar to conscious controls [78].

Directional connectivity, noninvasively measured, using multichannel EEG is a possible novel metric for assessing consciousness that is connected to the

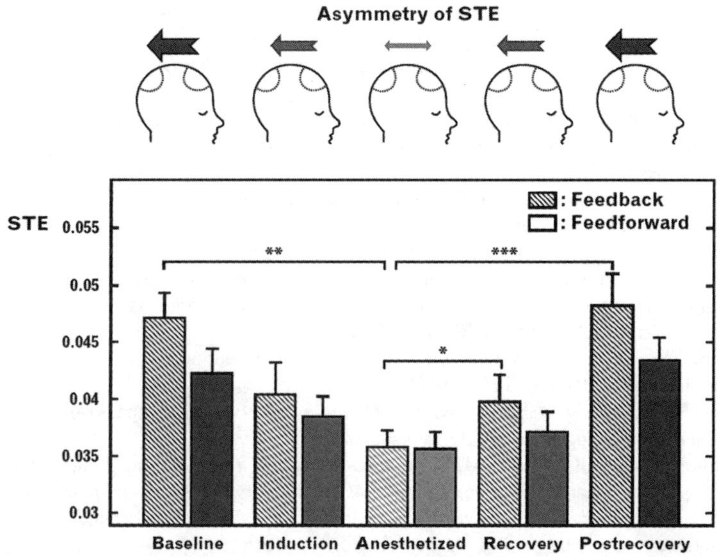

Fig. 1. Preferential inhibition of feedback connectivity (in striped bars) in the frontoparietal network. Note that at surgical anesthesia (*green*) with either propofol (n = 9) or sevoflurane (n = 9), both directions of frontal-parietal connectivity are suppressed. The measure of directional connectivity in this study was symbolic transfer entropy (STE) [74]. STE is one of several analytic techniques that assess causal interactions between the activity of 2 brain areas. Understanding the influence of one brain region on another allows us to infer the direction of information flow. (*From* Ku SW, Lee U, Noh GJ, et al. Preferential inhibition of frontal-to-parietal feedback connectivity is a neurophysiologic correlate of general anesthesia in surgical patients. PLoS One 2011;6:e251–55.)

environment. It is disrupted by different classes of anesthetics and in pathologic conditions, such as the vegetative state.

SUMMARY

Intraoperative awareness with explicit recall occurs in 1 to 2 cases per thousand and is linked to the neuroscientific problem of consciousness. Current brain monitoring techniques may be useful in preventing awareness during routine care or TIVA but are not superior to protocols based on anesthetic concentration. Real-time measure of functional and directional connectivity across different brain regions known to be important for connected consciousness may be the next wave of intraoperative brain monitors.

References

[1] Bigelow HJ. Insensibility during surgical operations produced by inhalation. Boston Med Surg J 1846;35:309–17.

[2] Rowan KJ. Awareness under TIVA: a doctor's personal experience. Anaesth Intensive Care 2002;34:505–6.

[3] Leslie K, Chan MT, Myles PS, et al. Posttraumatic stress disorder in aware patients from the B-aware trial. Anesth Analg 2010;110:823–8.

[4] Mashour GA, Orser BA, Avidan MS. Intraoperative awareness: from neurobiology to clinical practice. Anesthesiology 2011;114:1218–33.
[5] Hudetz AG. Are we unconscious during general anesthesia? Int Anesthesiol Clin 2008;46: 25–42.
[6] Crick F, Koch C. A framework for consciousness. Nat Neurosci 2003;6:119–26.
[7] Edelman G. The remembered present: a biological theory of consciousness. New York: Basic Books; 1990.
[8] Sanders RD, Tononi G, Laureys S, et al. Unresponsiveness ≠ unconsciousness. Anesthesiology 2012;116:946–59.
[9] Leslie K, Sleigh J, Paech MJ, et al. Dreaming and electroencephalographic changes during anesthesia maintained with propofol or desflurane. Anesthesiology 2009;111:547–55.
[10] Brice DD, Hetherington RR, Utting JE. A simple study of awareness and dreaming during anaesthesia. Br J Anaesth 1970;42:535–42.
[11] Sandin RH, Enlund G, Samuelsson P, et al. Awareness during anaesthesia: a prospective case study. Lancet 2000;355:707–11.
[12] Sebel PS, Bowdle TA, Ghoneim MM, et al. The incidence of awareness during anesthesia: a multicenter United States study. Anesth Analg 2004;99:833–9.
[13] Errando CL, Sigl JC, Robles M, et al. Awareness with recall during general anaesthesia: a prospective observational evaluation of 4001 patients. Br J Anaesth 2008;101:178–85.
[14] Davidson AJ, Smith KR, Blussé van Oud-Alblas HJ, et al. Awareness in children: a secondary analysis of five cohort studies. Anaesthesia 2011;66:446–54.
[15] Mashour GA, Esaki RK, Tremper KK, et al. A novel classification instrument for intraoperative awareness events. Anesth Analg 2010;110:813–5.
[16] Ghoneim MM, Block RI, Haffarnan M, et al. Awareness during anesthesia: risk factors, causes and sequelae: a review of reported cases in the literature. Anesth Analg 2009;108:527–35.
[17] Myles PS, Leslie K, McNeil J, et al. Bispectral index monitoring to prevent awareness during anaesthesia: the B-Aware randomised controlled trial. Lancet 2004;363:1757–63.
[18] American Society of Anesthesiologists Task Force on Intraoperative Awareness. Practice advisory for intraoperative awareness and brain function monitoring: a report by the American society of Anesthesiologists task force on intraoperative awareness. Anesthesiology 2006;104:847–64.
[19] Avidan MS, Zhang L, Burnside BA, et al. Anesthesia awareness and the Bispectral index. N Engl J Med 2008;358:1097–108.
[20] Flockhart D. Drug interactions: cytochrome P450 drug interaction table. Indiana University School of Medicine; 2007. Accessed May 21, 2012. Available at: http://medicine.iupui.edu/clinpharm/ddis/table.aspx.
[21] Liem EB, Lin CM, Suleman MI, et al. Anesthetic requirement is increased in redheads. Anesthesiology 2004;101:279–83.
[22] Cheng VY, Martin LJ, Elliott EM, et al. Alpha5GABAA receptors mediate the amnestic but not sedative-hypnotic effects of the general anesthetic etomidate. J Neurosci 2006;26:3713–20.
[23] Rau V, Oh I, Liao M, et al. Gamma-aminobutyric acid type A receptor β3 subunit forebrain-specific knockout mice are resistant to the amnestic effect of isoflurane. Anesth Analg 2011;113:500–4.
[24] Avidan MS, Jacobsohn E, Glick D, et al. Prevention of intraoperative awareness in a high-risk surgical population. N Engl J Med 2011;365:591–600.
[25] Zhang C, Xu L, Ma YQ, et al. Bispectral index monitoring prevent awareness during total intravenous anesthesia: a prospective, randomized, double-blinded, multi-center controlled trial. Chin Med J 2011;124:3664–9.
[26] Snow JD. On the inhalation of the vapour of ether in surgical operations. Br J Anaesth 1953;25:253–67, contd.
[27] Guedel AE. Inhalation anesthesia. 2nd edition. New York: Macmillan; 1951.
[28] Eger EI 2nd, Saidman LJ, Brandstater B. Minimum alveolar anesthetic concentration: a standard of anesthetic potency. Anesthesiology 1965;26:756–63.

[29] Bruhn J, Myles PS, Sneyd R, et al. Depth of anaesthesia monitoring: what's available, what's validated and what's next? Br J Anaesth 2006;97:85–94.
[30] Barnard JP, Bennett C, Voss LJ, et al. Can anaesthetists be taught to interpret the effects of general anaesthesia on the electroencephalogram? Comparison of performance with the BIS and spectral entropy. Br J Anaesth 2007;99:532–7.
[31] Bottros MM, Palanca BJ, Mashour GA, et al. Estimation of the bispectral index by anesthesiologists: an inverse turing test. Anesthesiology 2011;114:1093–101.
[32] Rampil IJ. A primer for EEG signal processing in anesthesia. Anesthesiology 1998;89: 980–1002.
[33] Viertiö-Oja H, Maja V, Sarkela M, et al. Description of the Entropy algorithm as applied in the Datex-Ohmeda S/5 Entropy Module. Acta Anaesthesiol Scand 2004;48:154–61.
[34] Schmidt GN, BISchoff P, Standl T, et al. Comparative evaluation of the Datex-Ohmeda S/5 Entropy Module and the BISpectral Index monitor during propofol-remifentanil anesthesia. Anesthesiology 2004;101:1283–90.
[35] Glass PS, Bloom M, Kearse L, et al. Bispectral analysis measures sedation and memory effects of propofol, midazolam, isoflurane, and alfentanil in healthy volunteers. Anesthesiology 1997;86:836–47.
[36] Liu J, Singh H, White PF. Electroencephalographic Bispectral index correlates with intraoperative recall and depth of propofol-induced sedation. Anesth Analg 1997;84: 185–9.
[37] Punjasawadwong Y, Boonjeungmonkol N, Phongchiewboon A. Bispectral index for improving anaesthetic delivery and postoperative recovery. Cochrane Database Syst Rev 2007;(4):CD003843.
[38] Hans P, Dewandre PY, Brichant JF, et al. Comparative effects of ketamine on Bispectral Index and spectral entropy of the electroencephalogram under sevoflurane anaesthesia. Br J Anaesth 2005;94:336–40.
[39] Barr G, Jakobsson JG, Owall A, et al. Nitrous oxide does not alter bispectral index: study with nitrous oxide as sole agent and as an adjunct to i.v. anaesthesia. Br J Anaesth 1999;82:827–30.
[40] Fahlenkamp AV, Peters D, Biener IA, et al. Evaluation of bispectral index and auditory evoked potentials for hypnotic depth monitoring during balanced xenon anaesthesia compared with sevoflurane. Br J Anaesth 2010;105:334–41.
[41] Whitlock EL, Villafranca AJ, Lin N, et al. Relationship between bispectral index values and volatile anesthetic concentrations during the maintenance phase of anesthesia in the B-Unaware trial. Anesthesiology 2011;115:1209–18.
[42] Niu J, Wang SJ, Zhang MZ, et al. The peak bispectral index time cannot predict early phase propofol pharmacodynamics with effect site-controlled infusion algorithm. Indian J Pharmacol 2012;44:41–5.
[43] Zanner R, Pilge S, Kochs EF, et al. Time delay of electroencephalogram index calculation: analysis of cerebral state, BISpectral, and Narcotrend indices using perioperatively recorded electroencephalographic signals. Br J Anaesth 2009;103:394–9.
[44] Kelz MB, Sleigh J. From the edge of oblivion: the dance between intrinsic neuronal currents and neuronal connectivity. Anesthesiology 2012;116:977–9.
[45] Kelz MB, Sun Y, Chen J, et al. An essential role for orexins in emergence from general anesthesia. Proc Natl Acad Sci U S A 2008;105:1309–14.
[46] Friedman EB, Sun Y, Moore JT, et al. A conserved behavioral state barrier impedes transitions between anesthetic-induced unconsciousness and wakefulness: evidence for neural inertia. PLoS One 2010;5:e11903.
[47] Palanca BJ, Mashour GA, Avidan MS. Processed electroencephalogram in depth of anesthesia monitoring. Curr Opin Anaesthesiol 2009;22:553–9.
[48] Scoville WB, Milner B. Loss of recent memory after bilateral hippocampal lesions. J Neurol Neurosurg Psychiatry 1957;20:11–21.
[49] Buzsáki G. Theta oscillations in the hippocampus. Neuron 2002;33:325–40.

[50] Perouansky M, Rau V, Ford T, et al. Slowing of the Hippocampal [theta] rhythm correlates with anesthetic-induced amnesia. Anesthesiology 2010;113:1299–309.
[51] Laureys S. The neural correlate of (un)awareness: lessons from the vegetative state. Trends Cogn Sci 2005;9:556–9.
[52] Tononi G. An information integration theory of consciousness. BMC Neurosci 2004;5:42.
[53] Tononi G. Consciousness, information integration, and the brain. Prog Brain Res 2005;150:109–26.
[54] Tononi G. Consciousness as integrated information: a provisional manifesto. Biol Bull 2008;215:216–42.
[55] Hudetz AG. Suppressing consciousness: Mechanisms of general anesthesia. Semin Anesth Perioperat Med Pain 2006;25:196–204.
[56] Lee U, Mashour GA, Kim S, et al. Propofol induction reduces the capacity for neural information integration: implications for the mechanism of consciousness and general anesthesia. Conscious Cogn 2009;18:56–64.
[57] Alkire MT, Haier RJ, Barker SJ, et al. Cerebral metabolism during propofol anesthesia in humans studied with positron emission tomography. Anesthesiology 1995;82:393–403 [discussion: 27A].
[58] Alkire MT, Haier RJ, Shah NK, et al. Positron emission tomography study of regional cerebral metabolism in humans during isoflurane anesthesia. Anesthesiology 1997;86:549–57.
[59] Veselis RA, Reinsel RA, Beattie BJ, et al. Midazolam changes cerebral blood flow in discrete brain regions: an H2(15)O positron emission tomography study. Anesthesiology 1997;87: 1106–17.
[60] Laureys S, Goldman S, Phillips C, et al. Impaired effective cortical connectivity in vegetative state: preliminary investigation using PET. Neuroimage 1999;9:377–82.
[61] Långsjö JW, Maksimow A, Salmi E, et al. S-ketamine anesthesia increases cerebral blood flow in excess of the metabolic needs in humans. Anesthesiology 2005;103: 258–68.
[62] Alkire MT, Haier RJ, Fallon JH. Toward a unified theory of narcosis: brain imaging evidence for a thalamocortical switch as the neurophysiologic basis of anesthetic-induced unconsciousness. Conscious Cogn 2000;9:370–86.
[63] Alkire MT, Miller J. General anesthesia and the neural correlates of consciousness. Prog Brain Res 2005;150:229–44.
[64] Velly LJ, Rey MF, Bruder NJ, et al. Differential dynamic of action on cortical and subcortical structures of anesthetic agents during induction of anesthesia. Anesthesiology 2007;107: 202–12.
[65] Mhuircheartaigh RN, Rosenorn-Lanng D, Wise R, et al. Cortical and subcortical connectivity changes during decreasing levels of consciousness in humans: a functional magnetic resonance imaging study using propofol. J Neurosci 2010;30:9095–102.
[66] Baars BJ. Global workspace theory of consciousness: toward a cognitive neuroscience of human experience. Prog Brain Res 2005;150:45–53.
[67] Boveroux P, Vanhaudenhuyse A, Bruno MA, et al. Breakdown of within- and between-network resting state functional magnetic resonance imaging connectivity during propofol-induced loss of consciousness. Anesthesiology 2010;113:1038–53.
[68] Liu X, Lauer KK, Ward BD, et al. Propofol disrupts functional interactions between sensory and high-order processing of auditory verbal memory. Hum Brain Mapp 2011; http://dx.doi.org/10.1002/hbm.21385.
[69] Ferrarelli F, Massimini M, Sarasso S, et al. Breakdown in cortical effective connectivity during midazolam-induced loss of consciousness. Proc Natl Acad Sci U S A 2010;107: 2681–6.
[70] Changeux J. Conscious processing: implications for general anesthesia. Curr Opin Anaesthesiol 2012;25:397–404.
[71] Lamme V, Roelfsema P. The distinct modes of vision offered by feedforward and recurrent processing. Trends Neurosci 2000;23:571–9.

[72] Murphy M, Bruno MA, Riedner BA, et al. Propofol anesthesia and sleep: a high-density EEG study. Sleep 2011;34:283A–91A.
[73] Murphy M, Riedner BA, Huber R, et al. Source modeling sleep slow waves. Proc Natl Acad Sci U S A 2009;106:1608–13.
[74] Lee U, Kim S, Noh GJ, et al. The directionality and functional organization of frontoparietal connectivity during consciousness and anesthesia in humans. Conscious Cogn 2009;18: 1069–78.
[75] Ku SW, Lee U, Noh GJ, et al. Preferential inhibition of frontal-to-parietal feedback connectivity is a neurophysiologic correlate of general anesthesia in surgical patients. PLoS One 2011;6:e25155.
[76] Boly M, Moran R, Murphy M, et al. Connectivity changes underlying spectral EEG changes during propofol-induced loss of consciousness. J Neurosci 2012;32:7082–90.
[77] Långsjö JW, Alkire MT, Kaskinoro K, et al. Returning from oblivion: imaging the neural core of consciousness. J Neurosci 2012;32:4935–43.
[78] Boly M, Garrido MI, Gosseries O, et al. Preserved feedforward but impaired top-down processes in the vegetative state. Science 2011;332:858–62.

Advances in Anesthesia 30 (2012) 29–46

ADVANCES IN ANESTHESIA

Carotid Artery Interventions and Anesthetic Technique

An Evidence-Based Review

Ryan P. Pong, MD*, Neil A. Hanson, MD

Department of Anesthesiology, Virginia Mason Medical Center, Mailstop B2-AN, 1100 Ninth Avenue, Seattle, WA 98101, USA

Keywords

• Carotid artery endarterectomy • Carotid artery stenting • Timing of surgery • Anesthetic technique • Regional • Perioperative complications

Key Points

- Patients with severe carotid disease are at high risk of suffering stroke, resulting in permanent debilitation or even death. Generally, patients are separated into two groups: those having symptomatic disease and those having asymptomatic disease.
- Large scientific trials seem to demonstrate that, in patients with symptomatic disease, carotid endarterectomy (CEA) is the treatment of choice offering benefit but bears a perioperative stroke and death rate of up to 7% in some studies [1–6]. With asymptomatic disease, patients are required to have severe-enough disease to warrant surgical intervention [7,8].
- Anesthetic techniques for CEA are also divided: regional and general categories. Advocates for regional anesthesia cite awake testing of central nervous system (CNS) function during carotid artery clamping as the reason this method should be superior to general anesthesia, which relies on indirect methods to ascertain cerebral blood flow. However, a large randomized trial has called into question the superiority of regional anesthetic techniques in improving outcomes for patients undergoing CEA [9].

INTRODUCTION

Stroke is the third leading cause of death in the United States and the leading cause of serious long-term disability [10]. Every year, approximately 795,000 people in the United States have a stroke, 87% of which are caused by an ischemic event [11]. An ischemic stroke can be caused by cardioembolic phenomena (20%),

Financial support: None.

*Corresponding author. *E-mail address*: Ryan.Pong@vmmc.org

0737-6146/12/$ – see front matter
http://dx.doi.org/10.1016/j.aan.2012.07.001

lacunar infarcts (30%), or atherothrombotic cardiovascular disease [12]. In North America and Europe, atherosclerosis of the arteries supplying the brain is a significant cause of ischemic stroke [13].

The pathologic condition by which extracranial carotid arteries narrow due to atherosclerosis is termed carotid artery stenosis. The significance of this narrowing is generally divided into moderate and severe subtypes. Studies have reported an annual stroke risk of approximately 2% to 5% for patients with asymptomatic severe carotid stenosis [14]. The prevalence of moderate asymptomatic carotid artery stenosis has been shown to be approximately 8%, whereas those patients with severe asymptomatic carotid artery stenosis are upwards of 3% of the general population (Table 1) [15]. These prevalence estimates increase with age and other risk factors, such as smoking, hypertension, diabetes, and hyperlipidemia.

As in coronary artery disease, the pathophysiology of stroke due to carotid artery disease is largely due to atherogenesis [16,17]. Factors such as dyslipidemia and uncontrolled hypertension cause a dramatic remodeling of native arteries, leading to noncompliant, narrow vessels that are prone to thrombus formation. Hypoperfusion through the narrowed carotid arteries may be the cause of a minority of ischemic strokes, whereas most seem to be a result from atherosclerotic plaque embolization or occlusion of the vessel secondary to thrombus [18].

AVAILABLE TREATMENTS

Patients with severe carotid disease are at high risk of suffering stroke, resulting in permanent debilitation or even death. They are defined as either having no symptoms despite proven pathology (asymptomatic) or have had a stroke or transient ischemic attacks (TIAs) in the past (symptomatic). Medical therapy is almost always instituted in the case of symptomatic carotid artery stenosis, involving some combination of antihypertensive therapy, platelet-inhibitors, and lipid-lowering drugs [19–22]. Two large trials also support surgical intervention in the setting of symptomatic carotid disease [2,3]. In the North American Symptomatic Carotid Endarterectomy Trial (NASCET), a portion of the study was terminated in 1991 after enrolling 659 patients with severe carotid stenosis (>70%). Investigators discovered that carotid endarterectomy (CEA) in these patients was associated with a 17% reduction of stroke risk at 2-years postoperatively and it was deemed unethical to continue to deny the benefits of CEA to those randomized to medical therapy alone. The European Carotid

Table 1
Stroke risk and CEA risk reduction

Degree of stenosis	Moderate (50%–70% stenosis)	Severe (>70% stenosis)
Prevalence-asymptomatic	8%	3%
Annual stroke risk	1%	2%–5%
CEA-risk reduction–symptomatic	—	17% at 2 y (NASCET) 11% at 3 y (ECST)

Surgery Trial (ECST) had similarly positive results. After enrolling 3024 patients and randomizing them to either medical therapy or surgical intervention, CEA seemed to confer an absolute risk reduction of 11.6% against stroke or death at 3 years. Again, this was only true if the patient had greater than 70% ipsilateral carotid artery stenosis. The average postoperative risk of stroke or death following surgery in both trials was approximately 7%. In the NASCET trial, for those symptomatic patients whose carotid stenosis was between 50% and 69%, the benefits of surgery were marginal as the 5-year absolute-risk reduction for any stroke or death was 7.7% compared with a 5-year risk of ipsilateral ischemic stroke or any perioperative stroke or death of 6.5%. This was further validated in a recent meta-analysis [23].

Evidence for surgical intervention in patients with asymptomatic carotid artery stenosis has been unclear because there have been very few large randomized controlled trials (RCTs). The Asymptomatic Carotid Artery Stenosis (ACAS) study [7] was the first large RCT published, and enrolled 1659 patients with greater than 60% stenosis. Patients were randomized to either surgery or aspirin and followed for a median of 2.7 years with the surgery itself carrying a 2.7% risk of stroke or death. Kaplan-Meier projections place the 5-year risk of stroke and/or death at 10.6% for the medical control group and 4.8% for the surgical intervention group. Interestingly, the degree of stenosis did not change outcome and the number of absolute deaths between groups was not significant. The European counterpart to ACAS, the Asymptomatic Carotid Surgery Trial [24] (ACST), enrolled 3120 patients with asymptomatic carotid artery stenosis greater than 60%. They had similarly positive findings, citing a 3.1% postsurgical risk of stroke or death, but showing a relative risk reduction of 50% with CEA over 5 years (from 12% in the medical arm to 6% in the surgical arm). Meta-analysis of these two large trials and others has called in to question the significance of these results [25,26]. When the data are pooled, it would seem that, although CEA has a relative risk reduction for stroke of up to 30% over 3 years, the absolute risk reduction is only 1% annually for the first few years after surgery. The marginal benefits of this intervention in asymptomatic patients need to be weighed against the 3% risk of perioperative death and stroke that accompany CEA.

Although CEA has long been considered to be the mainstay of interventional therapy for carotid artery disease, recently, less invasive methods of revascularization have been developed. These endovascular procedures have been gaining popularity for patients considered to be poor candidates for CEA [27]. Carotid artery stenting has largely replaced angioplasty and initially seemed promising as an alternative to surgery when the results of the Stenting and Angioplasty with Protection in Patients at High Risk for Endarterectomy (SAPPHIRE) trial [28] were released. Subsequent studies, however, showed that carotid artery stenting was associated with higher costs as well as increased risk of stroke and death [29–31]. This divergence may because patients enrolled in the SAPPHIRE trial were asymptomatic and subsequent studies enrolled high-risk symptomatic patients (Table 2).

Table 2
Compiled data conclusions

Trial	Date of publication	Outcomes	Conclusions
ECST	1998	Stroke or death	CEA is indicated for severe symptomatic carotid artery stenosis.
NASCET	1998	Stroke or death	CEA caused significant reduction in stroke with symptomatic severe stenosis (small reduction in events when stenosis was defined as moderate).
ACAS	1995	TIA, stroke, death	Asymptomatic patients with >60% stenosis are good candidates for CEA.
ACST	2004	Stroke or death	Asymptomatic patients with >70% stenosis gain a 50% relative reduction in stroke risk from CEA.
SAPPHIRE	2004	Stroke, death, MI	Carotid artery stenting is not inferior to CEA in patients with symptomatic stenosis (>50%) or asymptomatic stenosis (>80%)
SPACE	2006	Stroke, death, restenosis	Carotid artery stenting leads to greater rates of recurrent stenosis
ICSS	2010	Stroke, death, MI	Higher rates of death and stroke occurred in those patients undergoing carotid artery stenting
EVA-3S	2008	Stroke or death	Periprocedural risk of stroke or death was higher with carotid artery stenting

Abbreviations: MI, myocardial infarction; SPACE, Stenting-Supported Percutaneous Angioplasty of the Carotid Artery versus Endarterectomy; ICSS, International Carotid Stenting Study; EVA-3S, Endarterectomy versus Angioplasty in Patients with Symptomatic Severe Carotid Stenosis.

PERIOPERATIVE MANAGEMENT

Preoperative evaluation

Patients present for carotid revascularization on average at 62 to 66 years of age [2,3]. Therefore, several comorbidities affecting anesthetic considerations may be present. Specific risk factors have been identified that increase the risk for stroke or death. In the ECST, these include: presentation with cerebral TIA, female sex, systolic hypertension, and peripheral vascular disease [32]. Another study of more than 1100 surgeries found that more than two of the following were associated with an adverse event: age over 70, ipsilateral symptoms, severe hypertension (diastolic blood pressure >110 mm Hg), CEA preparing for coronary artery bypass graft, history of angina, evidence of internal carotid artery thrombus, and internal carotid artery stenosis near the carotid siphon [33]. Although much attention has gone into optimizing patient's chronic disease before surgery, the surgeon must weigh the time it takes for optimization against the risks of waiting to perform carotid revascularization: it has been shown to be most beneficial to have revascularization within 2 weeks of an ischemic event [34].

Neurologic examination
To benefit from carotid revascularization, patients must either have had a TIA, a stroke, or be at a significantly elevated risk of one (see previous discussion). Thus, patients that present for CEA include a large number of patients with damaged and or threatened neurologic tissue. A thorough neurologic history should be elicited and (at a minimum) a focused neurologic examination performed. Previous deficits, even though resolved, may reappear with sedation or residual anesthesia [35] and can be confused with a new deficit.

Cardiac
Carotid intima-media thickness, as a marker for atheromatous disease, has been used to refine coronary heart disease [36] risk because patients with carotid atheromatous disease are also likely to have concomitant coronary atheromatous disease. Patients with coronary artery disease, ideally, should be as optimized as possible on their medical regimen at time of surgery. Studies to evaluate myocardial function and at-risk myocardium, such as stress echocardiography or nuclear imaging studies, can be performed if they will change management [37]. If discovered, coronary artery disease that is amenable to revascularization presents an interesting dilemma: which surgery should be done first or should they be done concurrently? There are no definitive answers to this question because no well-designed studies have been performed. Only those with active acute coronary syndrome as well as cerebrovascular symptoms should undergo a synchronous revascularization of both the carotid and coronary arteries [38].

Hypertension
Several studies have found hypertension, either systolic (>180 mm Hg) [32] or diastolic (>110 mm Hg) [33] to be associated with increased risk of myocardial infarction (MI), stroke, or death. Efforts should be made preoperatively to control blood pressure, but there is no sound evidence to suggest that delaying surgery for blood pressure control will improve outcome. Current guidelines advocate antihypertensive therapy to maintain blood pressure less than 140/90 mm Hg [38]. In the period immediately surrounding a stroke, one must weigh the risk of hemorrhagic conversion at higher pressures versus inadequate perfusion at lower pressures. Perioperative blood pressure management during carotid revascularization is important and, therefore, determining a true baseline for the patient will be important for blood pressure targets (see later discussion).

Pulmonary
Pulmonary disease may also be present as an associated comorbidity and should be optimized before surgery. Because the time from stroke or TIA should be as short as possible, the surgeon must weigh the risk of waiting for medical optimization against the threat of recurrent neurologic injury. Specific note should be made of patients with pulmonary disease and planned regional anesthesia techniques. Although avoiding intubation in patients with a reactive airway component is laudable, the risk of anesthetizing the phrenic

nerve with either deep or superficial cervical plexus block needs consideration in those patients with chronic obstructive pulmonary disease and altered airway mechanics. Tobacco cessation is an important part of stroke prevention [39]. Smoking cessation at least 4 weeks before surgery reduces respiratory complications by 23% and greater than 8 weeks by 47%–a rate equal to that of nonsmokers [40]. There is some concern that, in the shorter term, smoking cessation could increase perioperative respiratory [41], myocardial [42], and cerebrovascular complications [43]. However, a recent meta-analysis failed to detect benefit or show harm for short-term smoking cessation [11,40].

Hematology

The antiplatelet drug, aspirin is a major part of medical therapy for occlusive cerebrovascular disease in preventing further ischemic events in those with prior symptoms [38]. The addition of dipyridamole or clopidogrel may occur based on multiple factors, including individual risk profile and cost [38]. Systemic anticoagulation is not typically indicated unless there are other extenuating features [38]. Lipid-lowering statins are usually prescribed to patients with TIA or stroke [38]. They have been shown to lower the incidence of subsequent stroke and coronary events [20,44].

Monitoring considerations

In addition to standard American Society of Anesthesiologists monitors, including a five-lead EKG to monitor for perioperative myocardial ischemia, an arterial line is usually placed either preinduction or postinduction, depending on the patient's comorbidities. This should aid in monitoring and treatment of blood pressure changes that can be both rapid and severe (see later discussion).

A great deal of energy has been expended creating numerous studies examining the merits of neurologic monitoring for carotid artery surgery. Possible modalities of monitoring are summarized in Table 3. The data are vast and confusing: no compelling data exist that mandate neurologic monitoring during CEA. Further, it is unclear which modality is best: an estimated 9000 patients would be necessary to demonstrate the success of one monitoring modality versus another [45].

The goal of neurologic monitoring is to detect cerebral ischemia secondary to hypoperfusion, thus signaling the need for an intervention, which may include raising arterial blood pressure or insertion of a shunt. A shunt is a small conduit that can be inserted proximal in the carotid artery, carrying blood around the site of the arteriotomy and endarterectomy to the distal internal carotid.

There is no standard practice surrounding the use of shunts [46]. Proponents of routine shunting espouse the benefits of preserving cerebral blood flow and allowing surgery to be done in an unhurried manner. Other surgeons may never shunt, citing reduced risk of dislodging plaque, thus reducing the embolic stroke risk and expediency of surgery limiting ischemic times in patients with compromised flow. Still others use shunts in a selective fashion based on neurologic monitoring [47]. A recent meta-analysis found that the risk of perioperative stroke with routine shunting was 1.4% compared with 2% for routine nonshunting. Selective shunting showed stroke rates from 1.1 to 4.8% depending on modality of neurologic monitoring [46]. In the light of inconclusive data [48], it seems that the best and most familiar practice for each surgeon and center should continue. However, knowledge of neurologic monitoring and how the effects of anesthesia potentially impact it needs to be understood by the anesthesia provider.

Anesthetic technique-general versus local

A large collaborative of investigators in 24 different countries began to look at whether the idea of regional anesthesia was actually better than general anesthesia for CEA [9]. This multicenter RCT enrolled 3526 subjects. The primary outcomes were: stroke, MI, or death within 30 days. Of these subjects, 93% in the "local" group received a cervical plexus block (deep or superficial), with 64% receiving supplementation by the surgeon during the operation. Though there were some differences between groups, there was no statistically significant difference in primary outcomes.

There were a few limitations to this study: (1) the intended sample size of 5000 subjects was not achieved and (2) higher-risk subjects avoided randomization altogether. The selection bias inherent in assigning higher risk subjects to one group because of clinical familiarity was more than likely necessary to achieve adequate patient recruitment and possibly provided better outcomes to the subjects. Unfamiliarity with certain methods of anesthesia by some of the investigators might have skewed the results in a similar manner if they had been forced to provide anesthesia they were uncomfortable with through the randomization process on subjects who were higher risk.

After this trial, a retrospective analysis of a large national surgical quality improvement program database (26,070) of CEA cases found that general anesthesia is an independent risk factor (overall odds ratio 2.18, 9% CI 1.17–4.04) for postoperative MI, particularly in patients with preoperative neurologic symptoms (odds ratio 5.41, 95% CI, 1.32–22.16) [49]. The choice of regional anesthesia or general anesthesia remains at the discretion of the individual centers and the surgical and anesthesiology staff. Whichever technique, local or general, is chosen, and whether associated neurologic monitoring is used or not, depends on the success rate of avoiding perioperative morbidity and mortality at that institution.

Anesthetic technique: regional

Advocates of regional anesthetic techniques for CEA surgery postulate that the neurologic monitoring of a conversant patient during carotid artery cross-clamp will provide early detection of inadequate cerebral perfusion [50], lower rates of shunting [51], lower cardiovascular morbidity, and shorter hospital stay [52]. To provide this anesthetic choice, two broad categories are available to the practitioner: peripheral nerve block (cervical plexus block) and neuraxial block (cervical epidural). In 2007, a large retrospective study was conducted to compare these two techniques in CEA surgery [53]. With 1828 surgeries analyzed in this study, the investigators noted a more than twofold rate of block failure and a significantly higher rate of life-threatening complications (2% compared with 0.3%) in the cervical epidural group. The largest RCT

Table 3
Summary of neuromonitoring modalities for carotid revascularization

	Modality	Considerations	Method	Failure rate
Function	Mental Status	• Requires awake patient, sedation may impair monitoring • Remote access to airway • Patient may become confused or combative with ischemia • Requires OR team dedicated to awake patient (sound level in OR and speed of surgery)	Awake patient—verbal conversation and motor function with squeaky toy frequently used	1.4% conversion to general anesthesia [9]
	EEG	• Measures cortical activity only • High false positive rate—cerebral slowing can be induced by anesthetic depth and hypothermia • May require a dedicated monitoring technician	Multiple electrode montage attached to patients scalp, passive EEG activity monitored	—
	BIS	• Simple to understand and use • Limited studies validating its use [71,72] and remains questionable [73,74] • Bilateral montage may be more useful [72]	Electrode montage attached to forehead, proprietary algorithm renders a BIS number	—

	SSEP	• Anesthetics affect signal quality [75] • Expensive, requires dedicated monitoring technician • Can detect subcortical ischemia (in contrast to EEG)	Peripheral stimulus delivered, latency and amplitude of cerebral activity measured	2%–5% [45,76] electrode placement or monitor failure
Flow	TCD	• Requires expertise using TCD equipment • Can detect emboli • Can detect cerebral hyperperfusion • Consensus of flow decrement to indicate shunting is debated [76]	2 MHz ultrasound probe fixed to head on middle cerebral artery, flow velocity monitored	21%–22% [45,76] mainly failure to find acoustic window to enable monitoring, also loss of probe position during surgery
	Stump pressure	• Simple, cheap • No consensus on pressure threshold [77,78] • Poor sensitivity [77]	After cross-clamping carotid, distal artery cannulated and pressure read via pressure transducer	—
Metabolism	NIRS	• Reading can be altered in various fashion by pressors (ephedrine vs phenylephrine) [79] • No consensus on threshold [80,81] • Poor specificity	Measure of cerebral regional oxygenation via sensor placed on forehead	2% [45] probe dislodgement

Abbreviaitons: BIS, bispectral analysis; EEG, electroencephalogram; NIRS, near-infrared spectroscopy; OR, operating room; SSEP, somatosensory evoked potential; TCD, transcranial doppler.

to date [9], which compares regional anesthesia to general anesthesia for CEA surgery, does not identify cervical epidural anesthesia as a local anesthetic technique. Instead, the investigators used cervical plexus block (both deep and superficial) as the definition (>93% of subjects). The increased risk of using cervical epidural anesthesia and the paucity of data in large RCTs signify that this article will focus on cervical plexus block as the preferred method of regional anesthesia. When discussing cervical plexus blocks, this technique is divided into two categories: deep and superficial. In order for either option to be successful, the anesthesiologist must be aware of the pertinent anatomy.

The cervical plexus is formed by the anterior divisions of the first four cervical nerve roots after exiting through their respective intervertebral foramen. The plexus, which is immediately posterior to the sternocleidomastoid muscle, divides into deep and superficial branches. The superficial cervical plexus supplies innervation to the skin of the neck, whereas the deep cervical plexus supplies the muscles beneath and in the diaphragm. The classic anatomic landmarks for either technique are the mastoid process, the transverse process of the sixth cervical vertebra, and the posterior border of the sternocleidomastoid muscle.

Deep cervical plexus

For the deep cervical plexus block, to estimate the insertion site of the needle, a line is drawn from the mastoid process to the transverse process of the sixth cervical vertebra, which is usually palpated at the level just below the cricoid cartilage. This line is then used to mark the transverse processes of C2, C3, and C4 by using fixed measurements caudal from the mastoid process itself. Either multiple smaller injections can be made at these three levels or a larger single injection can be made at C3.

Superficial cervical plexus

Blockade of the superficial cervical plexus, on the other hand, is much less involved. The same line used to connect the mastoid process and C6, which lies behind the posterior border of the sternocleidomastoid, is infiltrated subcutaneously with local anesthetic (Fig. 1). Both techniques can lead to the complications of infection, hematoma formation, the possibility of permanent nerve injury, and local anesthetic toxicity. However, the deep cervical plexus block is prone to higher instances of toxicity because of the proximity of injection near major vascular structures, blockade of the phrenic nerve, and even central neuraxial spread.

Given the potential higher risk inherent in the application of the deep cervical plexus block, it would logically follow that, when compared with superficial cervical plexus block, the deep cervical plexus block would have a lower failure rate when applied in the setting of CEA surgery. Pandit and colleagues [54] pooled the data of 83 papers to see if they could find any significant difference in these two types of cervical plexus block. There are some limitations to the study, given that the analysis was not strictly performed on only RCTs. However, the results are nonetheless surprising. Although there

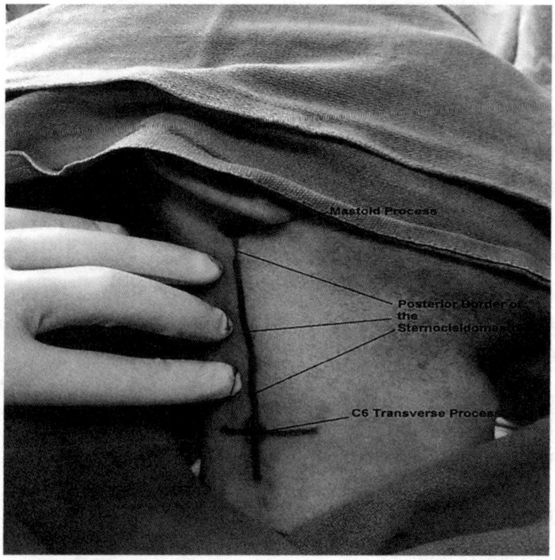

Fig. 1. Cervical plexus block surface anatomy.

was no significant difference between groups pertaining to all block-related complications, the deep cervical plexus group was twice as likely to have serious life-threatening complications. Another interesting discovery was that the deep cervical block group also was five times more likely to undergo conversion to general anesthesia. The two main reasons cited for conversion to general anesthesia were: (1) block failure and (2) anxiety of the patient. In either instance, most of those conversions occurred in the deep cervical plexus block group. Given this evidence, it would seem that if a regional anesthetic technique were to be used, the superficial cervical plexus block would provide the best outcome with the least amount of risk to the patient.

Anesthetic technique: general

Choice of drugs

No one anesthetic technique has been shown to be advantageous over another. There are several potential benefits to different anesthetic regimens, however. Using the newer, less soluble, inhaled anesthetics (desflurane and sevoflurane) may allow for a faster emergence [55,56], which facilitates obtaining an expeditious postoperative neurologic examination. The synthetic opioid remifentanil may have several potential benefits. These include suppression of cough, making emergence smoother, and a rapid, predictable offset [23] time due to the lack of context-sensitive half-time and minimal alveolar concentration–sparing effect (allowing hypnotic agents to be administered at decreased levels, which can contribute to faster emergence time). There is also great interest in using target-controlled infusions of remifentanil in conjunction propofol as part of total intravenous anesthetic technique to allow a hybrid anesthetic type of general anesthesia for opening and closing with emergence while remaining intubated and cooperative, with neurologic examination for the cross-clamping portion [57,58]. Nitrous oxide has been used in the past because of its low solubility leading to a favorable emergence profile as well as the potential hemodynamic it may offer. It does not cause as much hypotension as the other potent inhaled anesthetics can. There are some possible drawbacks, including (1) risk of air entrainment into the vascular system and the potential for nitrous oxide to expand that air [59] and (2) potential for cerebral activation, which is problematic in potentially ischemic areas of the brain [60].

The anesthesiologist may consider continued neuromuscular blockade, although it is not necessary to aid with surgical exposure. The depth of anesthesia needed for CEA is not great, especially if local anesthetic is used, and the lack neuromuscular blockade may predispose to patient movement and or coughing if a light plane of anesthesia is used.

Emergence

A rapid emergence helps facilitates the prompt diagnosis of operative complications that is immediately repairable, such as an intimal flap or thrombosis at the endarterectomy site. Coughing can increase blood pressure acutely. Avoidance of coughing may be prevented with intravenous lidocaine [61] (1.5–2 mg/kg) or by the anesthetic technique chosen; for instance, a potent rapid-acting opioid (remifentanil) [62] as an antitussive agent. In some centers, the operating room and back table are maintained sterilely until a neurologic examination is performed in case surgical reexploration is needed.

Intraoperative considerations

Blood pressure

The management of blood pressure during CEA varies depending on the phase of surgery. During initial dissection and carotid artery cross-clamp, blood pressure should be maintained at baseline or even elevated up to 20%. Because of the flow limitation introduced by the shunt (decreased radius and increased length of transit) augmenting pressure may allow for preservation of blood flow. Augmenting blood pressure in the patient without a shunt may allow for improved collateral flow during the potentially ischemic time. Elevating the blood pressure must be weighed against the risk of inducing ischemia by either the increase in afterload or inotropy necessary to achieve this goal [63]. After carotid revascularization, blood pressure should be maintained at normal or slightly lower than normal levels to prevent cerebral hyperperfusion syndrome (see later discussion).

Acute changes of blood pressure can be a signal for intraoperative complications. A carotid artery dissection, embolism, or hypoperfusion and/or ischemia may lead to hypertension. Bradycardia and hypotension during CEA are usually the result of direct stimulation of the carotid sinus, resulting in an erroneous interpretation of a hypertensive state inducing vagal outflow. This can be treated and prevented by anesthetizing the carotid sinus on the surgical field. This same effect can be seen during carotid stenting when the balloon dilation occurs.

Glycemic control

Patients with and without diabetes have been shown to have worse outcomes with hyperglycemia [64]. Neuronal tissue is sensitive to glucose levels and, if elevated, stimulate metabolism potentially leading to ischemia and cell death [65].

Carbon dioxide

Maintenance of normocapnia seems to be the most logical approach to ventilation. Hypercapnia leads to cerebral vasodilation. The areas distal to the blocked carotid artery, however, are likely to be maximally vasodilated with little vasomotor reserve. Therefore, in the setting of hypercapnia, vasodilation of normal areas of the brain occurs and may potentially steal blood away from the less perfused areas [66]. Conversely, hypocapnia may allow for the "Robin Hood effect" (vasoconstriction of the normal cerebral areas may direct blood toward the ischemic areas that are maximally vasodilated to begin with and are incapable of vasoconstriction to hypocapnia). Aggressive hyperventilation (hypocapnia), however, can induce decreased global cerebral blood flow, worsening areas with impaired circulation.

Postoperative considerations

Neck hematoma

A defect in arteriotomy closure or poor wound hemostasis may cause a neck hematoma, which can occur in 1.4% to 5.5% of patients and may be exacerbated by postoperative hypertension [67]. A hematoma may develop rapidly, leading to airway obstruction and the potential for difficult mask ventilation and/or intubation (40% of the time) [67]. The airway should be secured and the surgeon notified immediately. Emergent decompression of the hematoma may be necessary to allow tracheal intubation.

MI

Patients with carotid artery disease have proven vascular disease, thus, they are at high risk for having coexisting coronary artery disease. The proinflammatory state of surgery as well as attempts at increasing perfusion to the brain during the surgery may cause perioperative MI. The incidence of perioperative MI has been found to be 0.2 to 0.5% [9,49].

Hyperperfusion syndrome

The brain distal to the stenosis of the carotid artery has become accustomed to lower perfusion pressures. As the autoregulatory curve shifts to the right under chronic hypertensive conditions, there is a similar left shift in the autoregulatory curve of the hypoperfused tissue. After the carotid stenosis has been corrected, this tissue is acutely exposed to normal systemic pressures that can induce hyperperfusion in 12.5% of patients postoperatively. This pressure, even though it may be normal, may by too high for the tissue distal to the opened blockage and may lead to hyperperfusion syndrome (1.9%), which resembles severe hypertensive symptoms such as headache, cerebral edema, and seizures, and can lead to intracerebral hemorrhage (0.37%) [68]. These patients should continue to have invasive blood pressure monitoring with careful control for several days, allowing the autoregulatory mechanisms to normalize to the new, higher perfusing pressures.

Stroke

Despite using the most diligent care (shunting, monitoring, embolic protection devices) strokes may occur about 4% of the time [9]. Although much effort is made trying to monitor for adequate cerebral perfusion to prevent hypoperfusion ischemic strokes, most strokes are from embolism from the carotid plaque.

Other postoperative considerations

Cranial nerve palsies occur from surgical insult in approximately 5% cases [69,70]. Most commonly these are hypoglossal, vagus, or facial nerve branches and, less often, the laryngeal (superior and recurrent). Most cranial nerve palsies resolve with time. In the ECST, 4 months postoperatively, only 0.5% of cranial nerve injuries persisted [69].

SUMMARY

Carotid revascularization has been shown to be superior to medical therapy when the stenosis is symptomatic. Beyond this, much room is left for interpretation of the myriad of studies that deal with treatment of asymptomatic stenosis, including (1) the manner in which to revascularize, (2) carotid artery stenting versus open CEA, (3) whether to shunt or not to shunt, (4) whether to use neurologic monitoring (if so, which monitor to use), (5) anesthetic selection (general vs regional), and (6) which anesthetic agents to use (in the case of general anesthesia). When regional anesthesia is selected, a superficial cervical plexus block is the most efficacious technique with the least amount of risk. There is great latitude to devise the best practice and, for now, doing what is the most successful is appropriate. The stroke rate for a specific center and surgeon cannot be greater than that of doing maximal medical therapy. It is hopeful that ongoing studies and analyses will help shed light on what direction and refinements in protocols will allow the best possible outcome for these common procedures.

References

[1] Beneficial effect of carotid endarterectomy in symptomatic patients with high-grade carotid stenosis. North American Symptomatic Carotid Endarterectomy Trial Collaborators. N Engl J Med 1991;325:445–53.

[2] Barnett HJ, Taylor DW, Eliasziw M, et al. Benefit of carotid endarterectomy in patients with symptomatic moderate or severe stenosis. North American Symptomatic Carotid Endarterectomy Trial Collaborators. N Engl J Med 1998;339:1415–25.

[3] Randomised trial of endarterectomy for recently symptomatic carotid stenosis: final results of the MRC European Carotid Surgery Trial (ECST). Lancet 1998;351:1379–87.

[4] Rothwell PM, Slattery J, Warlow CP. Clinical and angiographic predictors of stroke and death from carotid endarterectomy: systematic review. BMJ 1997;315:1571–7.

[5] Hertzer NR, O'Hara PJ, Mascha EJ, et al. Early outcome assessment for 2228 consecutive carotid endarterectomy procedures: the Cleveland Clinic experience from 1989 to 1995. J Vasc Surg 1997;26:1–10.

[6] Earnshaw JJ. Carotid endarterectomy-the evidence. J R Soc Med 2002;95:168–70.

[7] Endarterectomy for asymptomatic carotid artery stenosis. Executive Committee for the Asymptomatic Carotid Atherosclerosis Study. JAMA 1995;273:1421–8.
[8] Benavente O, Moher D, Pham B. Carotid endarterectomy for asymptomatic carotid stenosis: a meta-analysis. BMJ 1998;317:1477–80.
[9] Lewis SC, Warlow CP, Bodenham AR, et al. General anaesthesia versus local anaesthesia for carotid surgery (GALA): a multicentre, randomised controlled trial. Lancet 2008;372: 2132–42.
[10] Heron M, Hoyert DL, Murphy SL, et al. Deaths: final data for 2006. Natl Vital Stat Rep 2009;57:1–134.
[11] Roger VL, Go AS, Lloyd-Jones DM, et al. Heart disease and stroke statistics—2011 update: a report from the American Heart Association. Circulation 2011;123:e18–209.
[12] Rosamond WD, Folsom AR, Chambless LE, et al. Stroke incidence and survival among middle-aged adults: 9-year follow-up of the Atherosclerosis Risk in Communities (ARIC) cohort. Stroke 1999;30:736–43.
[13] Lansberg MG, O'Donnell MJ, Khatri P, et al. Antithrombotic and thrombolytic therapy for ischemic stroke: antithrombotic therapy and prevention of thrombosis, 9th ed: American College of Chest Physicians Evidence-Based Clinical Practice Guidelines. Chest 2012;141:e601S–36S.
[14] Inzitari D, Eliasziw M, Gates P, et al. The causes and risk of stroke in patients with asymptomatic internal-carotid-artery stenosis. North American Symptomatic Carotid Endarterectomy Trial Collaborators. N Engl J Med 2000;342:1693–700.
[15] de Weerd M, Greving JP, Hedblad B, et al. Prevalence of asymptomatic carotid artery stenosis in the general population: an individual participant data meta-analysis. Stroke 2010;41:1294–7.
[16] Libby P, Theroux P. Pathophysiology of coronary artery disease. Circulation 2005;111: 3481–8.
[17] Golledge J, Greenhalgh RM, Davies AH. The symptomatic carotid plaque. Stroke 2000;31: 774–81.
[18] Sitzer M, Muller W, Siebler M, et al. Plaque ulceration and lumen thrombus are the main sources of cerebral microemboli in high-grade internal carotid artery stenosis. Stroke 1995;26:1231–3.
[19] Baigent C, Keech A, Kearney PM, et al. Efficacy and safety of cholesterol-lowering treatment: prospective meta-analysis of data from 90,056 participants in 14 randomised trials of statins. Lancet 2005;366:1267–78.
[20] Amarenco P, Bogousslavsky J, Callahan A 3rd, et al. High-dose atorvastatin after stroke or transient ischemic attack. N Engl J Med 2006;355:549–59.
[21] PROGRESS Collaborative Group. Randomised trial of a perindopril-based blood-pressure-lowering regimen among 6,105 individuals with previous stroke or transient ischaemic attack. Lancet 2001;358:1033–41.
[22] Halkes PH, van Gijn J, Kappelle LJ, et al. Aspirin plus dipyridamole versus aspirin alone after cerebral ischaemia of arterial origin (ESPRIT): randomised controlled trial. Lancet 2006;367:1665–73.
[23] Rothwell PM, Eliasziw M, Gutnikov SA, et al. Analysis of pooled data from the randomised controlled trials of endarterectomy for symptomatic carotid stenosis. Lancet 2003;361: 107–16.
[24] Halliday A, Mansfield A, Marro J, et al. Prevention of disabling and fatal strokes by successful carotid endarterectomy in patients without recent neurological symptoms: randomised controlled trial. Lancet 2004;363:1491–502.
[25] Chambers BR, Donnan GA. Carotid endarterectomy for asymptomatic carotid stenosis. Cochrane Database Syst Rev 2005;(4):CD001923.
[26] Guay J, Ochroch EA. Carotid endarterectomy plus medical therapy or medical therapy alone for carotid artery stenosis in symptomatic or asymptomatic patients: a meta-analysis. J Cardiothorac Vasc Anesth 2012 epub ahead of print, Available online 9 April 2012.

[27] Endovascular versus surgical treatment in patients with carotid stenosis in the Carotid and Vertebral Artery Transluminal Angioplasty Study (CAVATAS): a randomised trial. Lancet 2001;357:1729–37.

[28] Yadav JS, Wholey MH, Kuntz RE, et al. Protected carotid-artery stenting versus endarterectomy in high-risk patients. N Engl J Med 2004;351:1493–501.

[29] Ringleb PA, Allenberg J, Bruckmann H, et al. 30 day results from the SPACE trial of stent-protected angioplasty versus carotid endarterectomy in symptomatic patients: a randomised non-inferiority trial. Lancet 2006;368:1239–47.

[30] Mas JL, Chatellier G, Beyssen B, et al. Endarterectomy versus stenting in patients with symptomatic severe carotid stenosis. N Engl J Med 2006;355:1660–71.

[31] Ederle J, Dobson J, Featherstone RL, et al. Carotid artery stenting compared with endarterectomy in patients with symptomatic carotid stenosis (International Carotid Stenting Study): an interim analysis of a randomised controlled trial. Lancet 2010;375:985–97.

[32] Bond R, Narayan SK, Rothwell PM, et al. Clinical and radiographic risk factors for operative stroke and death in the European carotid surgery trial. Eur J Vasc Endovasc Surg 2002;23:108–16.

[33] McCrory DC, Goldstein LB, Samsa GP, et al. Predicting complications of carotid endarterectomy. Stroke 1993;24:1285–91.

[34] Rothwell PM, Eliasziw M, Gutnikov SA, et al. Endarterectomy for symptomatic carotid stenosis in relation to clinical subgroups and timing of surgery. Lancet 2004;363:915–24.

[35] Thal GD, Szabo MD, Lopez-Bresnahan M, et al. Exacerbation or unmasking of focal neurologic deficits by sedatives. Anesthesiology 1996;85:21–5 [discussion: 29A–30A].

[36] Nambi V, Chambless L, Folsom AR, et al. Carotid intima-media thickness and presence or absence of plaque improves prediction of coronary heart disease risk: the ARIC (Atherosclerosis Risk In Communities) study. J Am Coll Cardiol 2010;55:1600–7.

[37] Fleisher LA, Beckman JA, Brown KA, et al. ACC/AHA 2007 guidelines on perioperative cardiovascular evaluation and care for noncardiac surgery: a report of the American College of Cardiology/American Heart Association Task Force on Practice Guidelines (Writing Committee to revise the 2002 guidelines on perioperative cardiovascular evaluation for noncardiac surgery): developed in collaboration with the American Society of Echocardiography, American Society of Nuclear Cardiology, Heart Rhythm Society, Society of Cardiovascular Anesthesiologists, Society for Cardiovascular Angiography and Interventions, Society for Vascular Medicine and Biology, and Society for Vascular Surgery. Circulation 2007;116:e418–99.

[38] Brott TG, Halperin JL, Abbara S, et al. 2011 ASA/ACCF/AHA/AANN/AANS/ACR/ASNR/CNS/SAIP/SCAI/SIR/SNIS/SVM/SVS guideline on the management of patients with extracranial carotid and vertebral artery disease: executive summary: a report of the American College of Cardiology Foundation/American Heart Association Task Force on practice guidelines, and the American Stroke Association, American Association of Neuroscience Nurses, American Association of Neurological Surgeons, American College of Radiology, American Society of Neuroradiology, Congress of Neurological Surgeons, Society of Atherosclerosis Imaging and Prevention, Society for Cardiovascular Angiography and Interventions, Society of Interventional Radiology, Society of NeuroInterventional Surgery, Society for Vascular Medicine, and Society for Vascular Surgery. Stroke 2011;42:e420–63.

[39] Wolf PA, D'Agostino RB, Kannel WB, et al. Cigarette smoking as a risk factor for stroke. The Framingham Study. JAMA 1988;259:1025–9.

[40] Wong J, Lam DP, Abrishami A, et al. Short-term preoperative smoking cessation and postoperative complications: a systematic review and meta-analysis. Can J Anaesth 2012;59:268–79.

[41] Warner DO. Helping surgical patients quit smoking: why, when, and how. Anesth Analg 2005;101:481–7, table of contents.

[42] Ruiz-Bailen M, de Hoyos EA, Reina-Toral A, et al. Paradoxical effect of smoking in the Spanish population with acute myocardial infarction or unstable angina: results of the ARIAM Register. Chest 2004;125:831–40.
[43] Ovbiagele B, Saver JL. The smoking-thrombolysis paradox and acute ischemic stroke. Neurology 2005;65:293–5.
[44] Amarenco P, Goldstein LB, Sillesen H, et al. Coronary heart disease risk in patients with stroke or transient ischemic attack and no known coronary heart disease: findings from the Stroke Prevention by Aggressive Reduction in Cholesterol Levels (SPARCL) trial. Stroke 2010;41:426–30.
[45] Moritz S, Schmidt C, Bucher M, et al. Neuromonitoring in carotid surgery: are the results obtained in awake patients transferable to patients under sevoflurane/fentanyl anesthesia? J Neurosurg Anesthesiol 2010;22:288–95.
[46] Aburahma AF, Mousa AY, Stone PA. Shunting during carotid endarterectomy. J Vasc Surg 2011;54:1502–10.
[47] Pennekamp CW, Moll FL, de Borst GJ. The potential benefits and the role of cerebral monitoring in carotid endarterectomy. Curr Opin Anaesthesiol 2011;24:693–7.
[48] Bond R, Rerkasem K, Counsell C, et al. Routine or selective carotid artery shunting for carotid endarterectomy (and different methods of monitoring in selective shunting). Cochrane Database Syst Rev 2002:CD000190.
[49] Leichtle SW, Mouawad NJ, Welch K, et al. Outcomes of carotid endarterectomy under general and regional anesthesia from the American College of Surgeons' National Surgical Quality Improvement Program. J Vasc Surg 2012;56:81–8.
[50] Agrifoglio G, Bonalumi FA. Prediction of cerebral ischaemia using loco-regional anaesthesia. Eur J Vasc Endovasc Surg 1993;7(Suppl A):13–5.
[51] Benjamin ME, Silva MB Jr, Watt C, et al. Awake patient monitoring to determine the need for shunting during carotid endarterectomy. Surgery 1993;114:673–9 [discussion: 679–81].
[52] McCarthy RJ, Walker R, McAteer P, et al. Patient and hospital benefits of local anaesthesia for carotid endarterectomy. Eur J Vasc Endovasc Surg 2001;22:13–8.
[53] Hakl M, Michalek P, Sevcik P, et al. Regional anaesthesia for carotid endarterectomy: an audit over 10 years. Br J Anaesth 2007;99:415–20.
[54] Pandit JJ, Satya-Krishna R, Gration P. Superficial or deep cervical plexus block for carotid endarterectomy: a systematic review of complications. Br J Anaesth 2007;99:159–69.
[55] Umbrain V, Keeris J, D'Haese J, et al. Isoflurane, desflurane and sevoflurane for carotid endarterectomy. Anaesthesia 2000;55:1052–7.
[56] Kostopanagiotou G, Markantonis SL, Polydorou M, et al. Recovery and cognitive function after fentanyl or remifentanil administration for carotid endarterectomy. J Clin Anesth 2005;17:16–20.
[57] Bevilacqua S, Romagnoli S, Ciappi F, et al. Anesthesia for carotid endarterectomy: the third option. Patient cooperation during general anesthesia. Anesth Analg 2009;108:1929–36.
[58] Marcucci G, Siani A, Accrocca F, et al. Preserved consciousness in general anesthesia during carotid endarterectomy: a six-year experience. Interact Cardiovasc Thorac Surg 2011;13:601–5.
[59] Pasternak JJ, Lanier WL. Is nitrous oxide use appropriate in neurosurgical and neurologically at-risk patients? Curr Opin Anaesthesiol 2010;23:544–50.
[60] Reinstrup P, Ryding E, Ohlsson T, et al. Regional cerebral metabolic rate (positron emission tomography) during inhalation of nitrous oxide 50% in humans. Br J Anaesth 2008;100: 66–71.
[61] Gefke K, Andersen LW, Friesel E. Lidocaine given intravenously as a suppressant of cough and laryngospasm in connection with extubation after tonsillectomy. Acta Anaesthesiol Scand 1983;27:111–2.
[62] Lee JH, Koo BN, Jeong JJ, et al. Differential effects of lidocaine and remifentanil on response to the tracheal tube during emergence from general anaesthesia. Br J Anaesth 2011;106: 410–5.

[63] Boysen G, Engell HC, Ladegaard-Pedersen HJ, et al. Effect of induced hypertension on internal carotid artery stump pressure and rCBF during carotid surgery. Eur Neurol 1971;6:355–60.

[64] Nardi K, Milia P, Eusebi P, et al. Predictive value of admission blood glucose level on short-term mortality in acute cerebral ischemia. J Diabetes Complications 2012;26:70–6.

[65] Prakash A, Matta BF. Hyperglycaemia and neurological injury. Curr Opin Anaesthesiol 2008;21:565–9.

[66] Boysen G, Ladegaard-Pedersen HJ, Henriksen H, et al. The effects of PaCO2 on regional cerebral blood flow and internal carotid arterial pressure during carotid clamping. Anesthesiology 1971;35:286–300.

[67] Shakespeare WA, Lanier WL, Perkins WJ, et al. Airway management in patients who develop neck hematomas after carotid endarterectomy. Anesth Analg 2010;110:588–93.

[68] Moulakakis KG, Mylonas SN, Sfyroeras GS, et al. Hyperperfusion syndrome after carotid revascularization. J Vasc Surg 2009;49:1060–8.

[69] Cunningham EJ, Bond R, Mayberg MR, et al. Risk of persistent cranial nerve injury after carotid endarterectomy. J Neurosurg 2004;101:445–8.

[70] Assadian A, Senekowitsch C, Pfaffelmeyer N, et al. Incidence of cranial nerve injuries after carotid eversion endarterectomy with a transverse skin incision under regional anaesthesia. Eur J Vasc Endovasc Surg 2004;28:421–4.

[71] Estruch-Perez MJ, Ausina-Aguilar A, Barbera-Alacreu M, et al. Bispectral index changes in carotid surgery. Ann Vasc Surg 2010;24:393–9.

[72] Kodaka M, Nishikawa Y, Suzuki T, et al. Does bilateral bispectral index monitoring (BIS) detect the discrepancy of cerebral reperfusion during carotid endarterectomy? J Clin Anesth 2009;21:431–4.

[73] Dahaba AA; Xue JX, Hua Y, et al. The utility of using the bispectral index-Vista for detecting cross-clamping decline in cerebral blood flow velocity. Neurosurgery 2010;67:ons102–7 [discussion: ons107].

[74] Deogaonkar A, Vivar R, Bullock RE, et al. Bispectral index monitoring may not reliably indicate cerebral ischaemia during awake carotid endarterectomy. Br J Anaesth 2005;94: 800–4.

[75] Boisseau N, Madany M, Staccini P, et al. Comparison of the effects of sevoflurane and propofol on cortical somatosensory evoked potentials. Br J Anaesth 2002;88:785–9.

[76] Moritz S, Kasprzak P, Arlt M, et al. Accuracy of cerebral monitoring in detecting cerebral ischemia during carotid endarterectomy: a comparison of transcranial Doppler sonography, near-infrared spectroscopy, stump pressure, and somatosensory evoked potentials. Anesthesiology 2007;107:563–9.

[77] Hans SS, Jareunpoon O. Prospective evaluation of electroencephalography, carotid artery stump pressure, and neurologic changes during 314 consecutive carotid endarterectomies performed in awake patients. J Vasc Surg 2007;45:511–5.

[78] Moore WS, Hall AD. Carotid artery back pressure: a test of cerebral tolerance to temporary carotid occlusion. Arch Surg 1969;99:702–10.

[79] Nissen P, Brassard P, Jorgensen TB, et al. Phenylephrine but not ephedrine reduces frontal lobe oxygenation following anesthesia-induced hypotension. Neurocritic Care 2010;12: 17–23.

[80] Pennekamp CW, Bots ML, Kappelle LJ, et al. The value of near-infrared spectroscopy measured cerebral oximetry during carotid endarterectomy in perioperative stroke prevention. A review. Eur J Vasc Endovasc Surg 2009;38:539–45.

[81] Pedrini L, Magnoni F, Sensi L, et al. Is near-infrared spectroscopy a reliable method to evaluate clamping ischemia during carotid surgery? Stroke Res Treat 2012;2012:156975.

Advances in Anesthesia 30 (2012) 47–59

ADVANCES IN ANESTHESIA

Anesthetic Considerations in TEVAR and TAVI

Christopher M. Reidy, MD

Department of Anesthesiology, University of Wisconsin Hospital and Clinics, University of Wisconsin-Madison, 600 Highland Avenue, B6/319 CSC, Madison, WI 53792, USA

Keywords

• TEVAR • TAVI • Aortic aneurysm • Aortic stenosis • Anesthesia

Key Points

- Thoracic endovascular aortic repair (TEVAR) and transcatheter aortic valve implantation (TAVI) are state-of-the-art techniques for the treatment of thoracic aortic and aortic valve diseases.
- TEVAR and TAVI offer minimally invasive endovascular treatment alternatives to patients who have traditionally required major open surgical repair. These advances have reduced the risk of major surgical complications and extended the possibility of aortic repair to patients who suffer from advanced comorbidities.
- Anesthesiologists must understand these new techniques as they become more widely applied to provide optimal perioperative care, especially as the patient population changes to include an older and higher risk cohort.

INTRODUCTION

TEVAR and TAVI are state-of-the-art techniques for the treatment of thoracic aortic and aortic valve diseases. These techniques offer minimally invasive endovascular treatment alternatives to patients who have traditionally required major open surgical repair. These advances have reduced the risk of major surgical complications and extended the possibility of aortic repair to patients who suffer from advanced comorbidities. Anesthesiologists must understand these new techniques as they become more widely applied to provide optimal perioperative care, especially as the patient population changes to include an older and higher risk cohort. This article reviews current indications, procedural techniques, anesthetic management, and major complications of TEVAR and TAVI.

E-mail address: cmreidy@wisc.edu

0737-6146/12/$ – see front matter
http://dx.doi.org/10.1016/j.aan.2012.08.002

TEVAR

Procedure

TEVAR involves the placement of an endovascular stent graft into the thoracic aorta. Vascular access is obtained with delivery sheaths in the femoral or iliac arteries. A wire reinforced tube graft is delivered in retrograde fashion into the thoracic aorta. After appropriate positioning, as determined by angiography, the graft is deployed by inflating an endovascular balloon.

This procedure avoids the need for a large surgical incision, does not require one-lung ventilation or the placement of an aortic cross-clamp, and is rarely associated with significant bleeding. It imposes less hemodynamic stress on patients, and postoperative recovery is less complicated. TEVAR for aneurysmal disease requires suitable anatomy at the proximal and distal ends of the aneurysm to allow for transition between the stent graft and native aorta. Occasionally the stent graft covers the left subclavian artery, and in this case carotid-subclavian artery bypass may be necessary. If the graft extends into the abdominal aorta and covers visceral arteries, fenestrated or branched grafts are required.

Indications

Thoracic aortic aneurysm

TEVAR may be applied to aneurysms that involve the descending thoracic aorta. Thoracic aortic aneurysms (TAAs) involve only the thoracic aorta. Thoracoabdominal aortic aneurysms (TAAAs) involve both the thoracic and abdominal aorta. TAAAs are classified according to the Crawford system as types 1 through 4 [1]. Type 1 TAAAs originate in the proximal descending thoracic aorta and terminate above the renal arteries. TAAs and TAAAs traditionally required open surgical repair via thoracotomy or thoracoabdominal incision.

TEVAR was initially approved in 2005 for the elective endovascular repair of TAA after publication of a multicenter clinical trial [2]. TEVAR can also be used for repair of type 1 TAAAs. Endovascular repairs that extend father into the abdominal aorta require branched or fenestrated endografts and these techniques are being developed.

Type B aortic dissection

Thoracic aortic dissections can be classified according the Stanford system. Type A dissections involve the ascending aorta, and type B dissections involve only the descending aorta. Type B dissections are considered complicated if they are associated with organ malperfusion, contained rupture, or intractable pain despite optimal medical management.

Open surgical repair of acute complicated type B dissection is associated with a mortality rate as high as 50% [3]. TEVAR has been applied to patients with acute complicated type B dissections with a 30-day mortality rate of just 4% and improved 5-year survival compared with open repair [3].

Patients with uncomplicated type B dissections have traditionally been managed with medical therapy. The role of TEVAR in this population remains controversial. A randomized study comparing TEVAR with medical management showed no difference in 2-year survival or adverse events, despite a much higher rate of favorable aortic remodeling in the TEVAR group, perhaps because the study was underpowered [4].

Traumatic aortic injury
Most patients with thoracic aortic injuries resulting from blunt trauma die before reaching the hospital. Open surgical repair among survivors is associated with a 25% mortality rate and 16% paraplegia rate [5,6]. TEVAR has been applied as an off-label treatment in this setting. The extent of graft coverage required in this setting is typically small compared with aneurysms or dissections. The Society for Vascular Surgery, citing weak evidence, suggests that TEVAR is associated with improved survival and lower complication rates in these patients [6]

Complications
TEVAR was developed to reduce the significant morbidity and mortality associated with open surgical repair of the thoracic aorta. The most significant complications associated with thoracic aortic repair are death, spinal cord injury (SCI), and stroke.

Mortality
Mortality rates for elective surgical TAA and TAAA repair have improved over time, particularly at specialized high volume centers, which report mortality rates as low as 3% [7]. Experts consider this improvement to be the result of implementation of cerebrospinal fluid (CSF) drainage, therapeutic hypothermia, and improved hemodynamic management [7]. The overall risk of mortality nationally, however, is still estimated as high as 20%, with wide variation in reported rates [7,8].

Various studies show that elective TEVAR for TAA is associated with lower or equivalent mortality risk compared with open repair. The Gore TAG trial of TEVAR for TAA showed a procedural success rate of 98%, 30-day mortality rate of 1.5%, and 2-year mortality rate of 25% [2]. A retrospective nonrandomized comparison of elderly patients undergoing open repair or TEVAR showed 30-day mortality rates of 17% and 6% ($P = 0.1$), respectively, despite the presence of more severe comorbidities in the TEVAR group [9]. A large population-based analysis showed equivalent mortality rates (6%–7%) for open and endovascular repair despite more comorbidities in the TEVAR group [10].

Emergent TEVAR in the setting of ruptured TAA has a mortality rate of 48% [11].

Spinal cord injury
SCI is one of the most severe complications of thoracic or thoracoabdominal aortic repair. It results from interruption of spinal cord perfusion, causing ischemia and infarction. This may ultimately lead to immediate or delayed-onset paraplegia [12]. Reported rates of SCI after open surgical repair of all

TAAs and TAAAs range from 3% to 28% and may reflect variations in preoperative risk, extent of graft coverage, and differential application of spinal cord protective strategies [7,13].

TEVAR, despite its other advantages compared with open repair, can still lead to SCI. The etiology is multifactorial but probably includes interruption of spinal cord perfusion due to graft coverage of intercostal arteries [12–14]. Reimplantation of intercostal arteries is not possible with TEVAR.

The rate of SCI after TEVAR is 4% to 10% [1,12] even with selective use of CSF drainage catheters. The extent of graft coverage is the primary risk factor for SCI, with type 1 TAAA repairs conveying higher risk than TAA repairs [1,12]. The rate of SCI in isolated TAA repair is 1% for both open and endovascular repair [1]. The rate of SCI In type 1 TAAA repair is 10% for endovascular repair and 14% for open repair [1]. Prior distal aortic repair also increases the risk of paraplegia after TEVAR, as does involvement of the left subclavian artery [13]. Risk is increased because of interruption of collateral circulatory pathways.

Spinal cord protective strategies for both open and endovascular repair include CSF drainage, arterial pressure augmentation, hypothermia, and pharmacologic adjuncts, such as steroids, barbiturates, and naloxone [7]. CSF drainage and arterial pressure augmentation both serve to increase the spinal cord perfusion pressure gradient. Reimplantation of intercostal arteries and distal aortic perfusion may also be used during open repair.

Stroke

Risk factors for thoracic aortic disease are similar to those for cerebral vascular disease. Performance of TEVAR involves the placement wires and catheters into the proximal thoracic aorta and aortic arch, which may dislodge embolic debris. In one large series, more than half of the patients undergoing TEVAR had moderate or severe aortic atheroma. The risk of clinical stroke in this series was 5% [15]. In the multicenter Gore TAG trial, the stroke rate was 4% [2]. Proximal aortic coverage and intraoperative hypotension are associated with increased stroke risk [15].

Durability

Long-term durability of TEVAR compared with open repair remains unproved. Possible late complications include endoleak, device migration, and further aneurysm dilation [8]. Type 1 endoleak, which occurs when there is an incomplete seal at the end of the graft, is associated with early mortality after TEVAR [16].

Perioperative management

Anesthetic type

General, regional, and local (monitored anesthesia care) anesthetic techniques may be used for patients undergoing TEVAR. This decision should be based on individual patient conditions as well as institutional practice and familiarity.

General endotracheal anesthesia provides many advantages for the performance of TEVAR. It prevents patient movement and allows for precise control of ventilation, including intermittent apneic periods to facilitate angiography and device positioning. General anesthesia is necessary if deliberate moderate hypothermia is used for neuroprotection. A general anesthetic technique provides more control in the rare event that a major vascular complication mandates emergent conversion to open repair. It also allows for the use of transesophageal echocardiography (TEE).

Many centers routinely extubate patients in the operating room at the conclusion of the procedure. This is facilitated by the lack of incisional pain and rare need for massive fluid resuscitation. Emergence and extubation allow prompt performance of a neurologic examination. Extubation should not be attempted if a patient is hypothermic.

Regional or neuraxial anesthesia may also be used for select patients. Advantages may include faster recovery, avoidance of airway manipulation, less hemodynamic depression, and improved monitoring of mental status. Neuraxial blockade may confound a postoperative lower extremity neurologic examination and detection of SCI. Vasodilation associated with neuraxial block may reduce collateral spinal cord perfusion and could increase the risk of SCI.

Local anesthetic techniques are also useful in select cases. These include patients who are too hemodynamically unstable to tolerate general anesthesia. Local anesthesia also allows for continuous monitoring of lower extremity neurologic function in patients who are at high risk of SCI.

Regardless of technique, anesthetic management should allow for the maintenance and augmentation of aortic perfusion pressure because perioperative hypotension increases the risk of SCI [12].

Vascular access

Decisions regarding placement of vascular catheters should be based on the possible need for rapid resuscitation in the event of aortic rupture as well as the need for precise hemodynamic control to optimize spinal cord perfusion. Large-bore peripheral venous access is mandatory. All patients should have an arterial line placed for continuous blood pressure monitoring. If the left subclavian artery is involved in the repair, the arterial line should be placed in the right arm. A central venous line is routinely placed to facilitate administration of vasopressors and inotropes. A pulmonary artery catheter may be placed to measure cardiac output if a patient has significant myocardial dysfunction.

Transesophageal echocardiography

Intraoperative TEE may be used during the performance of TEVAR. Potential benefits include detection of aortic atheroma, confirmation of device position near the left subclavian artery, and guidance of hemodynamic support. Interposition of the trachea prevents imaging of the innominate and left common carotid arteries in most patients and interferes with imaging of the left subclavian in one-quarter of patients [17]. Placement of the probe in the esophagus may interfere with angiographic imaging. TEE should only be used by physicians who are qualified to interpret the images correctly and in patients for whom the benefits outweigh the risks of dysphagia and esophageal injury.

Evoked potential monitoring

Evoked potential monitoring is variably used during TEVAR to detect SCI. Early detection may allow for prompt interventions to improve spinal cord perfusion. These include CSF drainage (if a catheter is present), arterial blood pressure augmentation, or transfusion of red blood cells.

Monitoring strategies may include motor evoked potentials or somatosensory evoked potentials. Both are confounded to varying degrees by anesthetic technique, extremity hypoperfusion, and changes in depth of anesthesia. Motor evoked potentials provide a more direct assessment of anterior spinal cord perfusion, which is believed at increased risk because of perfusion from a single anterior spinal artery. Motor evoked potentials preclude the administration of neuromuscular blockade and are degraded by volatile anesthetics. Somatosensory evoked potentials are unaffected by neuromuscular blockade and less sensitive to volatile anesthetics, but they only monitor the posterior sensory tracts of the spinal cord.

Evoked potential monitoring may be a useful component of a multimodal strategy to detect and prevent SCI [13,14] during TEVAR; however, there are few clinical data to support its use [18].

CSF drainage

Perioperative management decisions for patients undergoing TEVAR must consider the risk of SCI. This risk depends on the extent of planned aortic repair as well as the integrity of collateral perfusion pathways. Assessment of this risk should be performed in collaboration with a vascular surgeon. There is limited evidence to guide decisions regarding CSF drainage for TEVAR. Clinical judgment must be used to weigh the potential benefit against the likelihood of complications associated with the procedure [14].

CSF drainage catheters may be placed to reduce CSF pressure. This increases the spinal cord perfusion pressure gradient and may reduce the incidence of SCI. Despite significant variation in study design, patient population, aneurysm extent, and management protocols, the available clinical evidence supports the use of CSF drainage to prevent or treat SCI during open TAAA repair [12,13]. A meta-analysis of 3 randomized controlled trials evaluating CSF drainage during open repair of types 1 and 2 TAAAs found that the number needed to treat to prevent SCI was 9 patients [19].

The risk of SCI after TEVAR for TAA and type 1 TAAA is 4% to 10%. The risk of SCI, when controlling for aneurysm type, is similar with open and endovascular repair in high-volume centers that use neuroprotective strategies. Preoperative placement of CSF drains should be considered more strongly in patients who at higher risk for SCI. Higher risk patients include those undergoing repair of type 1 TAAA (compared with isolated TAA) and those with prior distal aortic repair. CSF drainage may also be selectively implemented postoperatively if patients develop clinical evidence of SCI [20].

Patients undergoing TEVAR for traumatic aortic injury or plaque hemorrhage usually require a small area of graft coverage. The risk of SCI in this population is low and CSF drainage is rarely indicated.

Complications of CSF drainage include spinal headache, nerve root injury, cranial nerve palsy, neuraxial hematoma, intracranial hemorrhage, catheter fracture, and infection [12]. Catheter placement and removal must be performed when coagulation parameters are normal to reduce the risk of neuraxial hematoma. The risk of intracranial hemorrhage is increased when large volumes of CSF are drained rapidly. Analysis of a large single-center experience found that 0.2% of patients developed neuraxial hematoma, 3.5% developed intracranial hemorrhage, and 1% developed neurologic deficits attributable to CSF drainage [21].

Postoperative management

Immediate postoperative care of patients undergoing TEVAR should occur in a critical care unit. Providers must be able to promptly detect and manage complications including SCI, stroke, and hemorrhage. This includes the expertise to manage CSF drainage catheters and provide aggressive hemodynamic support. Established protocols and algorithms are recommended to facilitate prompt treatment of these complications because delay can severely compromise patient outcome.

TAVI

Procedure

TAVI refers to endovascular deployment of a bioprosthetic valve in the aortic position. A bioprosthetic valve is suspended within an expandable metal stent and deployed on the end of a delivery catheter. The procedure does not require sternotomy or cardiopulmonary bypass.

There are 2 types of valves currently in use [22]. The Edwards SAPIEN valve (Edwards Lifesciences, Irvine, California) has been approved for use in the United States and in Europe. This is a bovine bioprosthetic valve in a balloon-expandable stent. The Medtronic CoreValve (Medtronic, Minneapolis, Minnesota) is a porcine bioprosthetic valve suspended in a self-expanding stent. The CoreValve is currently approved only in Europe. A randomized trial of the CoreValve is under way in the United States.

Device access

Delivery access can be transfemoral or transapical (TA) depending on a patient's vascular anatomy [23]. TAVI is performed in most cases via the transfemoral route. The iliac or femoral artery is accessed in open or percutaneous fashion with delivery sheaths up to 24 French in diameter. Wire-guided catheters and the device are then advanced retrograde through the native aortic valve.

TF access is contraindicated in patients with severe vascular disease of the descending aorta or iliac arteries. In these patients, TAVI may be performed via the transapical route. A small left thoracotomy is made and the delivery sheath is inserted through the left ventricular apex. Catheters are then placed across the aortic valve in antegrade fashion. Transapical access is contraindicated by left ventricular apical thrombus.

Rapid ventricular pacing
Brief periods of rapid ventricular pacing to 200 beats per minute are required during the performance of TAVI [23,24]. Femoral venous access allows placement of a transvenous pacing wire into the right ventricle. Rapid pacing interrupts cardiac output and facilitates temporary occlusion of the aortic annulus during endovascular balloon inflation. This is required during balloon aortic valvuloplasty and valve deployment.

Balloon aortic valvuloplasty
Balloon aortic valvuloplasty of the native aortic valve is performed before deployment of the bioprosthetic valve. This facilitates leaflet separation in the heavily calcified and restricted native valve.

Device deployment
The prosthetic valve is collapsed and loaded on the tip of the delivery catheter. Device position within the aortic valve annulus is confirmed with angiography and TEE. The balloon is inflated and the stent is expanded. The native aortic valve leaflets are displaced to the side and provide traction for the newly implanted stent valve.

Confirmation of function
Immediately after deployment, the new valve is interrogated for proper function. It must be securely seated in the annulus without evidence of rocking or embolization. Normal leaflet motion should be visualized. The degree or intravalvular or paravalvular regurgitation must be determined.

Closure and hemostasis
The delivery apparatus is removed after confirmation of normal device function. Hemostasis must be obtained at the site of arterial vascular access. This may involve surgical closure of the iliac artery or the left ventricular apex depending on the approach used. Major bleeding or vascular injury may occur during this step.

Indications

TAVI is currently indicated for treatment of severe calcific aortic stenosis (AS) [24]. TAVI is not indicated for bicuspid aortic valves because the asymmetry of the aortic valve and root may prevent complete apposition of the stent and annulus. This could increase the risk of valve embolization or paravalvular regurgitation. TAVI is not indicated for primary aortic regurgitation. Currently available Edwards SAPIEN valves require that the annulus be between 18 mm and 25 mm in diameter.

TAVI was approved in the United States in 2011 for patients with severe AS who cannot undergo surgical aortic valve replacement (AVR) due to high operative risk. Surgical AVR has been recognized since 1982 to reduce mortality in patients with AS [25], and overall perioperative mortality rates are less than 3.2% [26]. Mortality rates, however, may exceed 10% to 30% in highly compromised patients [26,27]. Risk factors for increased mortality include diabetes, renal failure, lung disease, prior sternotomy, advanced heart failure, and old age [26]. As many as 30% of patients meeting indications for aortic or mitral valve replacement are denied surgery because of advanced comorbidities [28].

TAVI may one day provide a treatment alternative to reoperation for patients with degeneration of a surgically implanted bioprosthetic valve [24].

Complications

Mortality

TAVI was developed primarily to reduce the mortality rate of patients with severe AS and advanced comorbidities. Early data on TAVI were limited to small registries that showed periprocedural mortality rates between 6% and 12% [29]. Comparison with medical management or surgical AVR was based on historical controls or predicted operative mortality. The mortality rate associated with medical management of severe AS approaches 40% per year [30]. The predicted operative mortality rate for these patients based on risk models was approximately 15% to 30% [29]. These data were sufficient to gain device approval in Europe in 2007.

The landmark multicenter Placement of Aortic Transcather Valves (PARTNER) trial was performed between 2007 and 2010 [31,32]. This was the first randomized controlled evaluation of TAVI. There were 2 arms to this study. One arm included patients who were inoperable due to excessive mortality risk (≥50%). These patients were randomized to TAVI versus medical management, including balloon aortic valvuloplasty. The other arm included operable but high-risk patients (>10%–15% predicted mortality), and they were randomized to TAVI versus surgical AVR. Exclusion criteria in both arms included bicuspid aortic valve, need for coronary revascularization, ejection fraction less than 20%, recent stroke, or severe renal disease. It was sponsored by Edwards Lifesciences and used the Edwards SAPIEN valve.

The nonoperative arm showed superiority of TAVI compared with medical management [31]. The 1-year all-cause mortality rate for TAVI was 30% and for medical management was 50% ($P < .001$). The number needed to treat to prevent death was 5 and to prevent repeat cardiac related hospitalization was 3. The investigators concluded that TAVI is superior to medical management and should be considered standard of care for this population. The current Food and Drug Administration approval reflects this conclusion.

The operative arm of the study showed noninferiority of TAVI compared with AVR for high-risk patients [32]. The 30-day mortality rates for TAVI and AVR were 3% and 6%, respectively ($P = .07$). The 1-year all-cause mortality rates were 24% and 26%.

Stroke

Stroke is a major complication after TAVI. Most clinical strokes are due to procedure-related embolic events [24]. In TAVI, catheters are manipulated in the aortic root and ascending aorta with the risk of dislodging embolic debris. In one study, 84% of TAVI patients had evidence of embolic foci on brain MRI [33]. The rate of major stroke after TAVI is 4% to 8% [31,32]. This is higher than the stroke rate associated with AVR. TAVI-related stroke risk may improve with refinements in delivery systems and embolic protection devices.

Aortic regurgitation

Aortic regurgitation (AR) is a recognized complication after TAVI [23,24,31,32]. AR may be intravalvular or paravalvular. Mild AR occurs in 60% of TAVI procedures and is usually well tolerated.

Table 1
Incidence of aortic regurgitation after TAVI and AVR

	TAVI	AVR
Intravalvular AR		
Mild	62%	45%
Moderate–severe	1%	0%
Paravalvular AR		
Mild	60%	20%
Moderate–severe	7%	2%

Data from Smith CR, Leon MB, Mack MJ, et al. Transcatheter versus surgical aortic-valve replacement in high-risk patients. N Engl J Med 2011;364:2187–98.

Moderate or severe intravalvular AR is rare. It may result from overexpansion of the valve resulting in poor central leaflet coaptation or from one leaflet failing to close. Either of these problems may be treated by deploying a second prosthetic valve within the first. A stuck leaflet may also be released by gentle probing with a catheter. Intervention may need to be prompt because acute AR causes severe hemodynamic compromise.

Moderate or severe paravalvular AR occurs in 7% of TAVI cases. It has been associated with increased 1-year mortality [34]. Paravalvular AR results from incomplete apposition of the stent against the calcified and irregular endocardial surface of the aortic root. Repeated balloon expansion within the valve may lead to resolution of the problem.

Other complications

Other serious but rare complications associated with TAVI include prosthesis embolization, annular rupture, tamponade, coronary artery occlusion, mitral valve dysfunction, endocarditis, or vascular injury. Emergent institution of cardiopulmonary bypass or conversion to open surgery occurs less than 5% of the time [24,32]. The long-term durability of TAVI remains unproved.

Perioperative management

Logistic considerations

The perioperative approach to TAVI requires a unique degree of multidisciplinary collaboration between the cardiac surgeon, interventional cardiologist, anesthesiologist, echocardiographer, perfusionist, radiology assistants, and operating room nursing staff [24]. The procedure is performed in a hybrid operating room or modified catheterization laboratory. The room must be large enough to facilitate the aforementioned staff, have sophisticated angiographic capability, and allow for the emergent conversion to cardiopulmonary bypass.

Anesthetic type

TAVI can be performed with a variety of anesthetic techniques. All must address the hemodynamic fragility of patients with severe AS as well as the many comorbidities present in the TAVI patient population.

Standard management in the United States includes general endotracheal anesthesia [23,24]. This provides airway control, prevents patient movement, and accommodates intraoperative TEE. Single-lung ventilation is not necessary. Anesthetic management should allow for prompt extubation of patients in the operating room after completion of an uncomplicated procedure. Extubation is facilitated by maintenance with volatile anesthetics and remifentanil, avoidance of long acting opioids, and careful support of normothermia.

Perioperative management in Europe increasingly involves local and regional anesthetic techniques for transfemoral TAVI. These have been associated with shorter procedure time, less hemodynamic depression, shorter hospital length of stay, and equivalent mortality and procedural success rates [35]. This evolution in management has paralleled advances in procedural technique, equipment, and experience.

Vascular access

Standard of care in the United States currently involves placement of an arterial line, central venous line, pulmonary artery catheter, and large-bore peripheral venous catheters [24]. This reflects the possibility of severe procedural complications and the challenge of providing general anesthesia to patients with severe AS.

Hemodynamic management

Aggressive and precise hemodynamic management is required at all stages of TAVI, including induction, maintenance, and emergence. Prompt and adequate resuscitation from repeated episodes of rapid ventricular pacing is necessary to avoid cardiac arrest. Over-resuscitation, however, may lead to severe hypertension and serious bleeding, especially in transapical cases. This balance can be challenging in patients with hypertrophic dysfunctional ventricles.

Role of transesophageal echocardiography

Intraoperative TEE is routinely performed for TAVI in the United States [23,24]. The perioperative team includes a dedicated echocardiographer. This person may be a cardiologist or anesthesiologist who has no other competing responsibilities or tasks. TEE complements angiography and allows for intraoperative evaluation of aortic valve disease, annular size, device positioning, postdeployment valve function, hemodynamic status, and acute complications.

In Europe, the prevalence of local anesthetic techniques precludes routine use of TEE. Angiography is the primary tool for device positioning and evaluation of aortic regurgitation.

Postoperative management

TAVI patients should be managed postoperatively in a cardiac ICU by providers who are able to recognize and manage the complications of the procedure. Blood pressure and pain control are important considerations, especially for transapical patients. Early mobilization is encouraged. ICU length of stay is usually shorter for TAVI than for AVR. The average ICU length of stay in the PARTNER trial was 3 days [32]. Patients are treated for 6 months postoperatively with aspirin and clopidogrel [24].

References

[1] Greenberg RK, Lu K, Roselli EE, et al. Contemporary analysis of descending thoracic and thoracoabdominal aneurysm repair: a comparison of endovascular and open techniques. Circulation 2008;118:808–17.

[2] Makaroun MS, Dillavou ED, Kee ST, et al. Endovascular treatment of thoracic aortic aneurysms: results of the phase II multicenter trial of the GORE TAG thoracic endoprosthesis. J Vasc Surg 2005;41:1–9.

[3] Zeeshan A, Woo EY, Bavaria JE, et al. Thoracic endovascular aortic repair for acute complicated type B aortic dissection: superiority relative to conventional open surgical and medical therapy. J Thorac Cardiovasc Surg 2010;140:S109–15.

[4] Nienaber CA, Rousseau H, Eggebrecht H, et al. Randomized comparison of strategies for type B aortic dissection: the investigation of stent grafts in aortic dissection (INSTEAD) trial. Circulation 2009;120:2519–28.

[5] Ott MC, Stewart TC, Lawlor DK, et al. Management of blunt thoracic aortic injuries: endovascular stents versus open repair. J Trauma 2004;56:565–70.

[6] Lee WA, Matsumura JS, Mitchell RS, et al. Endovascular repair of traumatic thoracic aortic injury: clinical practice guidelines of the Society for Vascular Surgery. J Vasc Surg 2011;53: 187–92.

[7] Acher C, Wynn M. Outcomes in open repair of the thoracic and thoracoabdominal aorta. J Vasc Surg 2010;52:3S–9S.

[8] Gutsche JT, Szeto W, Cheung AT. Endovascular stenting of thoracic aortic aneurysm. Anesthesiol Clin 2008;26:481–99.

[9] Patel HJ, Williams DM, Upchurch GR, et al. A comparison of open and endovascular descending thoracic aortic repair in patients older than 75 years of age. Ann Thorac Surg 2008;85:1597–604.

[10] Orandi BJ, Dimick JB, Deeb GM, et al. A population-based analysis of endovascular versus open thoracic aortic aneurysm repair. J Vasc Surg 2009;49:1112–6.

[11] Geisbusch P, Kotelis D, Weber TF, et al. Endovascular repair of ruptured thoracic aortic aneurysms is associated with high perioperative mortality and morbidity. J Vasc Surg 2010;51: 299–304.

[12] Fedorow CA, Moon MC, Mutch AC, et al. Lumbar cerebrospinal fluid drainage for thoracoabdominal aortic surgery: rationale and practical considerations for management. Anesth Analg 2010;111:46–58.

[13] Sinha AC, Cheung AT. Spinal cord protection and thoracic aortic surgery. Curr Opin Anaesthesiol 2010;23:95–102.

[14] Cheung AT, Pochettino A, McGarvey ML, et al. Strategies to manage paraplegia risk after endovascular stent repair of descending thoracic aortic aneuryms. Ann Thorac Surg 2005;80:1280–9.

[15] Feezor RJ, Martin TD, Hess PJ, et al. Risk factors for perioperative stroke during thoracic endovascular aortic repairs (TEVAR). J Endovasc Ther 2007;14:568–73.

[16] Khoynezhad A, Donayre CE, Smith J, et al. Risk factors for early and late mortality after thoracic endovascular aortic repair. J Thorac Cardiovasc Surg 2008;135: 1103–9.

[17] Cheung AT, Gutsche JT, Moeller PJ, et al. Anatomic constraints to transesophageal echocardiographic imaging of the aortic arch branch vessels. Anesthesiology 2007;107:A1319.
[18] Weigang E, Hartert M, Siegenthaler MP, et al. Perioperative management to improve neurologic outcome in thoracic or thoracoabdominal stent grafting. Ann Thorac Surg 2006;82: 1679–87.
[19] Cina CS, Abouzahr L, Arena GO, et al. Cerebrospinal fluid drainage to prevent paraplegia during thoracic and thoracoabdominal aortic aneurysm surgery; a systematic review and meta-analysis. J Vasc Surg 2004;40:34–44.
[20] Keith CJ, Passman MA, Carignan MJ, et al. Protocol implementation of selective postoperative lumbar spinal drainage after thoracic endograft. J Vasc Surg 2012;55:1–9.
[21] Wynn MM, Mell MW, Tefera G, et al. Complications of spinal fluid drainage in thoracoabdominal aortic aneurysm repair: a report of 486 patients treated from 1987 to 2008. J Vasc Surg 2009;49:29–35.
[22] Klein AA, Webb ST, Tsui S, et al. Transcatheter aortic valve insertion: anaesthetic implications of emerging new technology. Br J Anaesth 2009;103:792–9.
[23] Billings FT, Kodali SK, Shanewise JS. Transcatheter aortic valve implantation: anesthetic considerations. Anesth Analg 2009;108:1453–62.
[24] Holmes DR Jr, Mack MJ, Kaul S, et al. 2012 ACCF/AATS/SCAI/STS expert consensus document on transcatheter aortic valve replacement. J Am Coll Cardiol 2012; http://dx.doi.org/10.1016/j.jacc.2012.01.001.
[25] Schwarz F, Baumann P, Manthey J, et al. The effect of aortic valve replacement on survival. Circulation 1982;66:1105–10.
[26] O'Brien SM, Shahian DM, Filardo G, et al. STS 2008 cardiac surgery risk models: part 2-isolated valve surgery. Ann Thorac Surg 2009;88:S23–42.
[27] Edwards FH, Peterson ED, Coombs LP, et al. Prediction of operative mortality after valve replacement surgery. J Am Coll Cardiol 2001;37:885–92.
[28] Iung B, Baron G, Butchart EG, et al. A prospective survey of patients with valvular heart disease in Europe: the Euro heart survey on valvular heart disease. Eur Heart J 2003;24: 1231–43.
[29] Zajarias A, Cribier AG. Outcomes and safety of percutaneous aortic valve replacement. J Am Coll Cardiol 2009;53:1829–36.
[30] Varadarajan P, Kapoor N, Bansal RC, et al. Clinical profile and natural history of 453 nonsurgically managed patients with severe aortic stenosis. Ann Thorac Surg 2006;82: 2111–5.
[31] Leon MB, Smith CR, Mack MJ, et al. Transcatheter aortic-valve implantation for aortic stenosis in patients who cannot undergo surgery. N Engl J Med 2010;363:1597–607.
[32] Smith CR, Leon MB, Mack MJ, et al. Transcatheter versus surgical aortic-valve replacement in high-risk patients. N Engl J Med 2011;364:2187–98.
[33] Kahlert P, Knipp SC, Schlamann M, et al. Silent and apparent cerebral ischemia after percutaneous transfemoral aortic valve implantation: a diffusion-weighted magnetic resonance imaging study. Circulation 2010;121:870–8.
[34] Tamburino C, Capodanno D, Ramondo A, et al. Incidence and predictors of early and late mortality after transcatheter aortic valve implantation in 663 patients with severe aortic stenosis. Circulation 2011;123:299–308.
[35] Dehedin B, Guinot PG, Ibrahim H, et al. Anesthesia and perioperative management of patients who undergo transfemoral transcatheter aortic valve implantation: An observational study of general versus local/regional anesthesia in 125 consecutive patients. J Cardiothorac Vasc Anesth 2011;25:1036–43.

Advances in Anesthesia 30 (2012) 61–73

ADVANCES IN ANESTHESIA

Continuous Peripheral Nerve Blocks for Pediatrics

Ravi Shah, MD*, Amod Sawardekar, MD,
Santhanam Suresh, MD

Department of Pediatric Anesthesiology, Ann & Robert H. Lurie Children's Hospital of Chicago, Feinberg School of Medicine, Northwestern University, 225 East Chicago Avenue, Box 19, Chicago, IL 60611, USA

Keywords

- Continuous peripheral nerve blockade • Pediatric regional anesthesia
- Peripheral nerve catheter • Nerve stimulation
- Ultrasound-guided regional anesthesia

Key Points

- Continuous peripheral nerve blocks (CPNBs) are gaining popularity in pediatrics with the advanced use of ultrasonography as well as accepted techniques of nerve stimulation [1].
- As more appropriate equipment has become available, a growing number of reports of their use for continuous postoperative pain management or therapeutic care in children have been published [2]. Most indications for continuous nerve blocks are for children undergoing procedures that are associated with significant or prolonged postoperative pain [3].
- CPNBs have also been reported as effective in both controlling pain and facilitating physical therapy in children with chronic regional pain syndromes [4].
- Despite such reports, limited data exist regarding the feasibility, safety, and efficacy of CPNB in children [5].

INDICATIONS

Indications for continuous peripheral nerve block (CPNB) include surgery associated with significant or prolonged postoperative pain, including major orthopedic surgery such as congenital hand or foot malformation repair; osteotomies of the humerus, femur, or tibia; limb-lengthening procedures; club foot repair; and femoral shaft fracture repair. In addition, postoperative pain management for several days after knee or ankle arthrolysis and knee ligamentoplasty may warrant placement of CPNB [2].

*Corresponding author. *E-mail address*: rdshah@luriechildrens.org

0737-6146/12/$ – see front matter
http://dx.doi.org/10.1016/j.aan.2012.09.001 Published by Elsevier Inc.

TECHNIQUES

Various techniques are currently used to place perineural catheters in children. Because indwelling catheters are left in place for some time, aseptic technique is mandatory. Nonstimulating catheter techniques have been described by Steele and colleagues [6] and a stimulating catheter technique has been described by Boezaart and colleagues [7]. The nonstimulating catheter technique involves placement of a conduit needle (ie, Tuohy needle or angiocatheter) near a nerve under ultrasound guidance or nerve stimulation. Saline or local anesthetic solution is then injected to expand the perineural space and a standard epidural catheter is advanced through the conduit needle using a modified Seldinger technique. The stimulating catheter technique uses an insulated conduit needle that is inserted in a similar fashion. A catheter with an electrically conductive connection to its tip is inserted through the conduit needle while stimulating the nerve (via the catheter) to ensure accurate positioning. A paucity of literature comparing these techniques remains within the pediatric literature. We commonly use both of these techniques at our institution with good results.

COMPLICATIONS AND ADVERSE SIDE EFFECTS

Complications of perineural catheters for continuous nerve blockade in adults are rare and less likely than those for single-injection nerve blocks [8]. Large comparative studies in this area have not been performed in children but several case reports suggest similar findings in the pediatric population [5]. Common problems associated with continuous nerve blockade are technical issues such as failed blocks, incomplete analgesia, catheter dislodgement, and leakage around the catheter entry site. More serious complications include infection, nerve injury, and systemic drug toxicity secondary to intravascular catheter placement or overdosage.

INFUSION STRATEGIES

The growing use of continuous regional anesthetic techniques in adults has led to a more prevalent use of CPNBs in the pediatric population [9]. Nerve anatomy in children (smaller diameters, short distances between the nodes of Ranvier) warrant large volumes and low concentrations of local anesthetic solution [10,11]. Despite this, a higher risk of toxicity exists in infants because of immature metabolic systems and lower albumin and α1-glycoprotein levels. Use of low-concentration L-enantiomer solutions (ropivicaine or levobupivacation) have been recommended for children because they are accompanied by low plasma concentrations, limiting the risk of local anesthetic systemic toxicity.

CPNBs FOR UPPER LIMB SURGERY

Infraclavicular approach to the brachial plexus

Indications

CPNBs are particularly useful for surgical procedures of the elbow, forearm, and hand. Perineural catheter placement via the axillary approach has been described in children with promising results with respect to pain control; however, difficulty in maintaining both immobilization and catheter sterility present significant limitations [12]. The infraclavicular approach to the brachial plexus does not present these limitations and is easier to perform for upper limb trauma when arm abduction is painful to perform. Continuous infraclavicular nerve blockade has been described in children as a safe and effective means to control perioperative acute pain after simplified skin fixation and radial osteotomy [13].

Technique

The brachial plexus cords are situated just inferior to the coracoid process. The axillary artery and vein lie medial to the cords, whereas the pectoralis major and minor are superficial to the neurovascular bundle. The lateral cord is visualized on ultrasound as a hyperechoic structure and the posterior cord is positioned deep to the axillary artery. The medial cord may be difficult to identify because of its anatomic location between the axillary artery and vein (See Fig. 1).

Marhofer and colleagues [14] described an approach to ultrasound-guided infraclavicular blockade in children using a lateral approach. The ultrasound probe is positioned in a transverse orientation below the clavicle to visualize the brachial plexus. An out-of-plane technique is used to advance the needle after it is inserted inferior to the probe. De Jose Maria and colleagues [15] placed the probe parallel to the clavicle in a parasagittal plane and directed the needle in a cephalad direction toward the brachial plexus. Catheter placement may be performed by either a nonstimulating or stimulating techniques. The catheter is checked for inadvertent intravascular placement and secured to the chest.

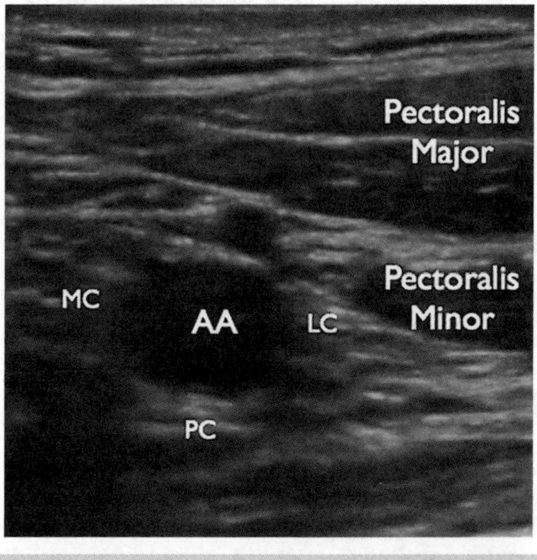

Fig. 1. Ultrasound image of the brachial plexus from the infraclavicular approach. The posterior, medial, and lateral cords surround the axillary artery.

Complications

Complications include hematoma, infection, nerve injury, and intravascular injection. The risk of a pneumothorax exists because of the proximity of the cervical pleura.

Postoperative care

For moderately painful upper limb surgery, continuous infraclavicular nerve blocks have significantly reduced pain and opioid requirements and increased patient satisfaction [16]. In adults, the combination of a continuous local anesthetic infusion with boluses is shown to provide optimal analgesia in this setting while minimizing oral analgesics compared with basal or bolus-only regimens [17]. However, this approach may not apply to younger children who are unable to appropriately administer demand doses.

Supraclavicular approach to the brachial plexus

Indications

The supraclavicular block provides analgesia for the upper arm and elbow. Indications for supraclavicular catheter placement include humeral osteotomy, humeral elongation, trauma, and arthrolysis [2]. De Jose Maria and colleagues [15] showed a higher success rate (without pneumothorax or Horner syndrome) with supraclavicular catheter placement in children compared with an infraclavicular approach.

Technique

Few techniques have been described in the pediatric population [15]. Nerve stimulation has not been recommended in children because of the increased risk of pneumothorax [18–20]. Ultrasound guidance is recommended rather than nerve stimulation to decrease this risk [15]. For block placement, the ultrasound probe is positioned in the coronal-oblique plane superior to the upper border of the

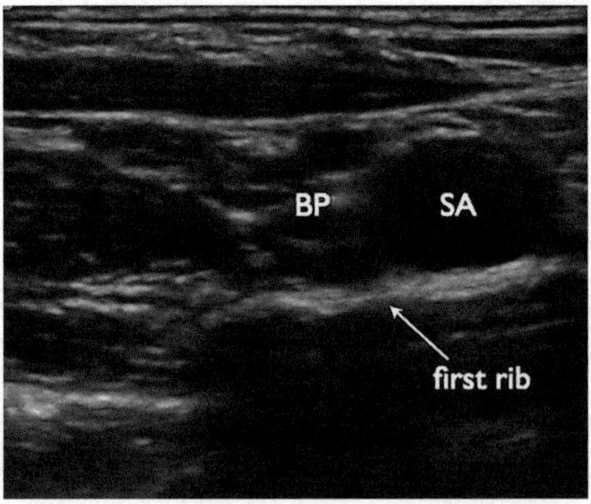

Fig. 2. Ultrasound image of the brachial plexus from the supraclavicular approach. The plexus lies superior and lateral to the subclavian artery and above the first rib.

midclavicle. The subclavian artery is visualized as a hypoechoic and pulsatile structure. An in-plane approach is used to direct the needle in a lateral-to-medial direction toward the brachial plexus, superior and lateral to the subclavian artery and above the first rib (See Fig. 2). Directing the needle in a lateral-to-medial direction avoids vascular structures and decreases the risk of intraneural injection. For continuous infusion, a 19-gauge or 20-gauge flexible epidural catheter may be placed through an introducer needle and advanced 1 to 3 cm beyond the needle tip between the brachial plexus and subclavian artery. The needle is removed over the catheter, the injection port is affixed, and the catheter is secured and test dosed.

Complications

Complications include hematoma, infection, hematoma, and intravascular injection. Furthermore, performing a supraclavicular block presents an increased risk of a pneumothorax because the lung parenchyma lies just medial to the first rib at the level where the block is completed. For this reason, visualization of the tip and shaft of the needle with ultrasonography may aid in its prevention.

Postoperative care

Despite the known efficacy of single-injection supraclavicular nerve blocks, limited data exist regarding continuous supraclavicular blocks and infusion strategies in children [21]. CPNB with supraclavicular catheters are typically used to provide 2 to 3 days of postoperative analgesia for pain related to upper extremity procedures.

Interscalene approach to the brachial plexus

Indications

The interscalene block provides analgesia to the shoulder and proximal arm via the trunks and roots of the brachial plexus that lie deep to the sternocleidomastoid (SCM) muscle and are surrounded by the anterior and middle scalene muscles. The C5, C6, and C7 nerve roots are visualized between the anterior and middle scalene muscles. This block is commonly performed for pediatric patients undergoing surgical procedures involving the shoulder or proximal humerus.

Only a few case reports have been published on the safety and feasibility of interscalene brachial plexus catheter placement for shoulder surgery in children and adolescents. CPNB at the interscalene level has been successfully used in children to manage postoperative pain after tumor resection from the cephalic end of the humerus [22]. The interscalene block is known for the risk of pneumothorax, vascular punctures, or epidural blockade. Ultrasound-guided interscalene catheter placement has been described in children as an easier and safer alternative to using nerve stimulation, resulting in fewer complications when performed by experienced practitioners [23].

Technique

The ultrasound probe is placed at the level of the cricoid cartilage at the posterolateral aspect of the SCM in the transverse oblique plane. Deep to the

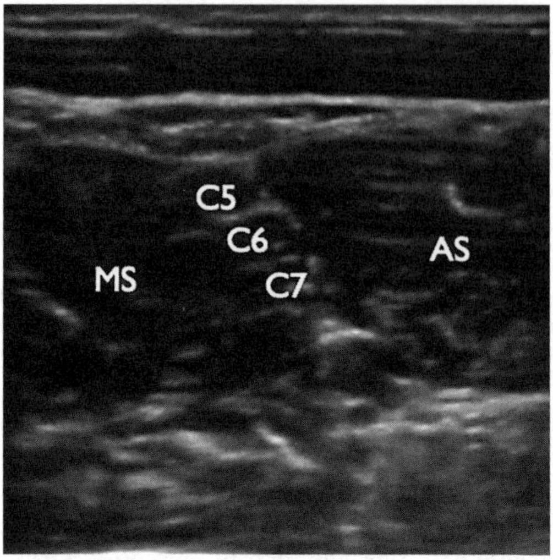

Fig. 3. Ultrasound image of the brachial plexus from the interscalene approach. The C5, C6, and C7 nerve roots are visualized between the anterior and middle scalene muscles.

SCM and lateral to the subclavian artery, the anterior and medial scalene muscles make up the interscalene groove. A hyperechoic structure contained within this region is the neurovascular bundle of the C5, C6, and C7 nerve roots (See Fig. 3). A catheter may be placed with ultrasound guidance in this region and secured at the skin. Although nerve stimulation may be used to deliver local anesthetic to the brachial plexus at this level, use of ultrasonography may decrease the total amount of local anesthetic required [6,7].

Complications

Block success is accompanied by hemidiaphragmatic paralysis, recurrent laryngeal nerve block, and Horner syndrome, so these should not be mistaken for complications [15,22]. The interscalene block should be used with caution in the pediatric population because of the potential risks of pneumothorax, vertebral artery injection, and intrathecal injection [24]. Ultrasound-assisted interscalene catheter placement is possible in children but is best performed by experienced clinicians [22].

CPNBs FOR ABDOMINAL SURGERY

Transversus abdominis plane block and continuous catheters

Indications

The transversus abdominis plane (TAP) block provides analgesia to the anterior abdominal wall, delivering postoperative analgesia but not surgical anesthesia [25]. Three muscle layers lie lateral to the rectus abdominus: the external oblique, internal oblique, and transversus abdominis. The thoracolumbar nerve roots(T8–L1) lie within the space (TAP plane) between the internal oblique and transversus abdominis muscle. These nerves provide sensory innervation to the muscles and skin of the anterior abdominal wall [8,26].

A single-shot TAP block with local anesthetic solution under ultrasound guidance is frequently used for pain management after abdominal incisions in combination with a systemic opioid regimen. The TAP block can be perpetuated by use of a catheter and continuous analgesia can be achieved with a local anesthetic infusion or bolus doses, thereby decreasing supplemental systemic opioid consumption [25].

Despite the paucity of data on the use of continuous TAP catheters in pediatric patients, this technique can provide a useful alternative to neuraxial analgesia. Unilateral TAP catheters have been successfully used in low-weight children for analgesia following single-sided open lower abdominal surgery when epidural analgesia was undesirable [27]. Similar reports have suggested that TAP catheters can provide excellent postoperative analgesia in patients with pre-existing neurologic deficits and severe spinal deformities via the administration of low-dose, low-concentration local anesthetic infusions [28].

Technique

Various techniques have been described that use an in-plane approach with ultrasound guidance, allowing needle advancement and the placement of local anesthetic in the TAP plane [25,29]. The ultrasound probe is positioned lateral to the umbilicus and moved lateral to the rectus abdominus to visualize the 3 muscle layers of the abdominal wall [30] (See Fig. 4). The needle is advanced using an in-plane technique to the TAP plane. Injection of local anesthetic creates an elliptical pocket of local anesthetic that the nerves traverse. For

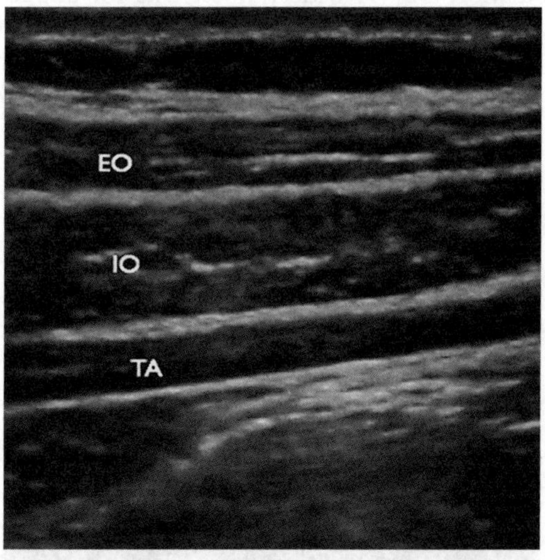

Fig. 4. Sonoanatomy of the transversus abdominus plane. Muscle layers include external oblique (EO), internal oblique (IO), and transversus abdominus (TA).

TAP catheter placement, a Tuohy-tip needle may be passed under ultrasound guidance using a similar in-plane approach and is placed between the transversus abdominis and internal oblique muscles. The tip of the catheter is localized sonographically by injecting local anesthetic or saline solution through the needle. The TAP plane is then expanded by injecting local anesthetic solution, which facilitates passage of an epidural catheter approximately 2 to 4 cm beyond the tip of the needle. The bevel of the needle is placed laterally to direct catheter migration in a lateral fashion. After test dose administration, the catheter can be secured by subcutaneous tunneling.

Complications

Intravascular injection, peritoneal and/or bowel puncture, and infection are potential complications of TAP catheter placement.

CPNBs FOR LOWER LIMB SURGERY

Continuous femoral nerve block

Indications

The femoral nerve block is primarily indicated for pain control in children for surgery of the femur (femoral shaft fractures, femoral tumor excision, and limb-lengthening procedures) or for surgical procedures involving the knee. The femoral nerve originates from nerve roots L2, L3, and L4 and provides analgesia from the anterior thigh to the knee when blocked. The nerve is located lateral to the femoral artery and vein, and can be visualized when the ultrasound probe is placed in the inguinal crease [31].

Continuous femoral nerve blocks have been used safely and effectively in the pediatric population [32]. A wide range exists for applicability, including use in children with cancer-related pain, CRPS, and acute postoperative pain.

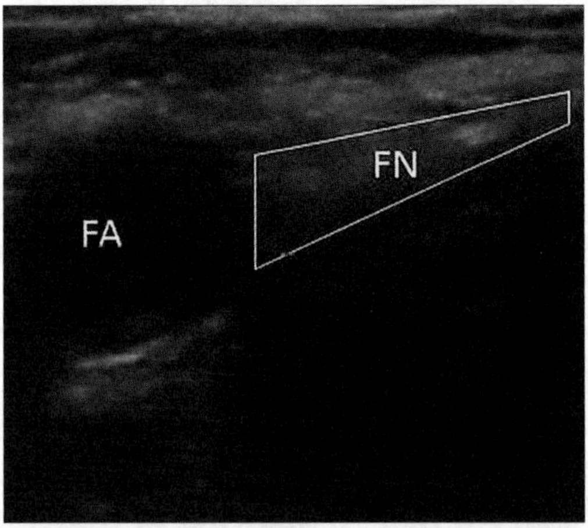

Fig. 5. Ultrasound image of the femoral nerve at the inguinal crease.

Technique

The patient is placed in the supine position and the femoral artery is located within the inguinal crease. When using nerve stimulation, the needle is advanced in a lateral-to-medial direction to elicit a quadriceps muscle twitch or patellar movement. Often there is thigh twitching indicating stimulation of the sartorius muscle, which should not misinterpreted as quadriceps stimulation. When using ultrasonography, the femoral vein, artery, and nerve can be visualized from medial to lateral (See Fig. 5). An in-plane or out-of-plane approach is used to direct needle placement to the femoral nerve to circumferentially surround it with local anesthetic [33,34].

For ultrasound-guided perineural catheter placement, an insulated Tuohy needle and a catheter with an inner steel spring that is capable of conducting electrical impulses to its distal tip (stimulating catheter) may be used. The needle tip is sonographically guided deep to the fascia iliaca and within the femoral nerve sheath. Placement may be confirmed by injecting saline or local anesthetic solution. A nerve stimulator clip is then attached to the proximal end of the stimulating catheter and the catheter is inserted into the needle. The catheter is advanced beyond the tip of the needle while simultaneously appreciating patellar movement with nerve stimulation. The catheter may be tunneled and secured, and should be test dosed before a bolus dose or infusion is started.

Complications

The femoral nerve's proximity to the vein and artery make vessel puncture and hematoma formation possible complications. Risks of indwelling catheter placement include infection and prolonged sensory blockade.

Continuous sciatic nerve block

Indications

Pain management for major foot and ankle surgery in children can be accomplished by continuous sciatic nerve block. Common pediatric indications include pain control for club foot repair, trauma, ankle osteosynthesis and exostosis, tibial and fibular osteotomy, and foot or toe amputation [35]. Continuous sciatic nerve blockade has been shown to have fewer adverse effects compared with epidural anesthesia in children undergoing major foot and ankle surgery [36]. The sciatic nerve is formed by nerve roots L4 to S3 and provides innervation to the posterior thigh and all but the medial aspect of the leg that lies distal to the knee. The sciatic nerve exits the pelvis in the greater sciatic foramen and courses inferior to the gluteus maximus muscle. The sciatic nerve continues to the posterior popliteal fossa then bifurcates to form the tibial and common peroneal nerves. The sciatic nerve can be blocked at the subgluteal, anterior thigh, or popliteal approaches in children. In addition, the use of continuous sciatic nerve blockade has been successfully described to provide extended analgesia [37,38]. Sciatic nerve catheter placement can be accurately and efficaciously facilitated with ultrasonography in children [39].

Technique

The sciatic nerve catheter can be placed at different locations (ie, subgluteal, anterior, or distal approach).

When approaching the sciatic nerve from the subgluteal area, the child is placed in a lateral decubitus position with the hip and knee flexed. The use of the ultrasonography allows nerve visualization between the greater trochanter and the ischial tuberosity deep to the gluteus maximus muscle. Both in-plane and out-of-plane approaches have been described with success. Nerve stimulation may be used alone or in conjunction with ultrasonography. When used, hamstring, calf, foot, and toe twitches are anticipated. Successful continuous nerve blockade with catheter placement at this level has been described in children [40].

The anterior approach to the sciatic nerve is executed by placing the patient in the supine position and using ultrasonography and/or nerve stimulation [41,42]. After the child is positioned supine, the leg is abducted and rotated laterally and the knee is flexed to the frog-leg position as the ultrasound probe is positioned below the inguinal crease. The sciatic nerve is seen deep and medial to the femur. This approach can be technically difficult in older children because of the increased depth to the sciatic nerve.

The distal approach in the popliteal fossa is the most frequently described in the pediatric literature. This approach is easy to perform and shows excellent quality and duration of analgesia with low doses of local anesthetic [43]. The patient is placed prone and the ultrasound probe is placed above the popliteal

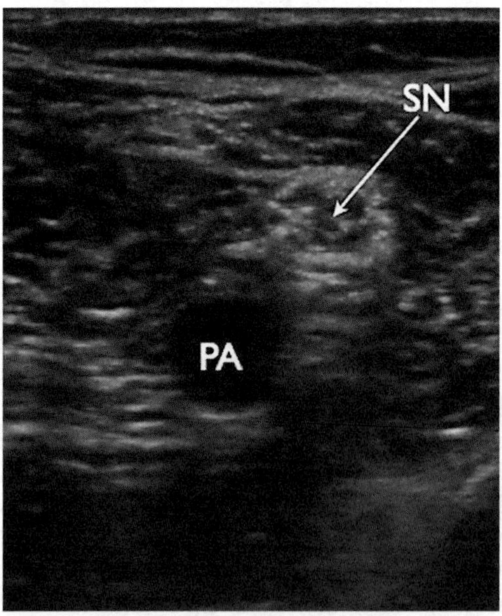

Fig. 6. Ultrasound image of the sciatic nerve from the distal approach in the popliteal fossa.

crease. The sciatic nerve is seen adjacent to the easily visualized popliteal artery (See Fig. 6). Moving distally, the tibial and common peroneal nerves can be seen separating from the sciatic nerve and may be blocked specifically. With the use of nerve stimulation, calf, foot, or toe twitches may be elicited at this location. As an alternative, the patient may remain in the supine position with the hip and knee flexed and the popliteal fossa approached using the same technique. Catheter insertion may be performed with stimulating or nonstimulating catheter approaches.

Complications

Complications include infection at the site of skin puncture and catheter placement, hematoma from vessel puncture, and local anesthetic toxicity. Compared with continuous epidural block in children undergoing major foot and ankle surgery, both techniques were associated with good postoperative analgesia, but children with continuous popliteal nerve catheters showed less urinary retention, less discontinuation of local anesthetic infusion, and less nausea and vomiting [2].

SUMMARY

CPNBs are emerging as an effective analgesic modality for children and can significantly contribute to an improved perioperative course by decreasing postoperative pain duration and intensity. The safety and ease of these techniques will likely facilitate early ambulation with improved rehabilitation.

References

[1] Tsui B, Suresh S. Ultrasound imaging for regional anesthesia in infants, children, and adolescents: a review of current literature and its application to neuraxial blocks. Anesthesiology 2010;112:719–28.

[2] Dadure C, Capdevila X. Peripheral catheter techniques. Paediatr Anaesth 2012;22: 93–101.

[3] Diwan R, Lakshmi V, Shah T, et al. Continuous axillary block for upper limb surgery in a patient with epidermolysis bullosa simplex. Paediatr Anaesth 2001;11:603–6.

[4] Dadure C, Motais F, Ricard C, et al. Continuous peripheral nerve blocks at home in the treatment of complex regional pain syndrome in children. Anesthesiology 2005;102:387–91.

[5] Ganesh A, Rose J, Wells L, et al. Continuous peripheral nerve blockade for inpatient and outpatient postoperative analgesia in children. Anesth Analg 2007;105(5):1234–42.

[6] Steele SM, Klein SM, D'Ercole FJ, et al. A new continuous catheter delivery system [letter]. Anesth Analg 1988;87:28.

[7] Boezaart AP, de Beer JF. Accurate placement of a catheter for selective continuous interscalene brachial plexus nerve block [abstract V14]. Sydney, Australia: World Congress of Anesthesiologists; 1996.

[8] Zaric D, Boysen K, Christiansen J, et al. Continuous popliteal sciatic nerve block for outpatient foot surgery: a randomized controlled trial. Acta Anaesthesiol Scand 2004;48:337–41.

[9] Ivani G, Tonetti F. Postoperative analgesia in infants and children: new developments. Minerva Anestesiol 2004;70:399–403.

[10] Bosenberg A, Ivani G. Regional anaesthesia: children are different [editorial]. Paediatr Anaesth 1998;8:447–50.

[11] Ilfeld BM, Morey TE, Wang RD, et al. Continuous popliteal sciatic nerve block for postoperative pain control at home. Anesthesiology 2002;97:959–65.

[12] Diwan R, Raux O, Troncin R, et al. Continuous infraclavicular brachial plexus block for acute pain management in children. Anesth Analg 2003;97:691–3.
[13] Ponde VC. Continuous infraclavicular brachial plexus block: a modified technique to better secure catheter position in infants and children. Anesth Analg 2008;106:94–6.
[14] Marhofer P. Upper extremity peripheral blocks. Tech Reg Anesth Pain Manag 2007;11: 215–21.
[15] De José María B, Banus E, Navarro EM, et al. Ultrasound-guided supraclavicular vs infraclavicular brachial plexus blocks in children. Paediatr Anaesth 2008;18:838–44.
[16] Ilfeld BM, Morey TE, Wright TW, et al. Interscalene perineural ropivicaine infusion: a comparison of two dosing regimens for postoperative analgesia. Reg Anesth Pain Med 2004;29:9–16.
[17] Ilfeld BM, Morey TE, Enneking FK. Infraclavicular perineural local anesthetic infusion: a comparison of three dosing regimens for postoperative analgesia. Anesthesiology 2004;100:395–402.
[18] Dalens B. Proximal blocks of the upper extremity: benefit/risk ratio. Regional anaesthesia in infants, children and adolescents. Baltimore (MD): Williams & Wilkins; 1995. p. 275–314.
[19] Tsui B, Suresh S. Ultrasound imaging for regional anesthesia in infants, children, and adolescents: a review of current literature and its application in the practice of extremity and trunk blocks. Anesthesiology 2010;112:473–92.
[20] Neal J, Brull R, Chan V. The ASRA evidence-based medicine assessment of ultrasound-guided regional anesthesia and pain medicine: executive summary. Reg Anesth Pain Med 2010;35:S1–9.
[21] Mariano E, Sandhu NS, Loland V, et al. A randomized comparison of infraclavicular and supraclavicular continuous peripheral nerve blocks for postoperative analgesia. Reg Anesth Pain Med 2011;36(1):26–31.
[22] Fredrickson MJ. Ultrasound-assisted interscalene catheter placement in a child. Anaesth Intensive Care 2007;35:807–8.
[23] Renes SH, Retting HC, Gielen MJ, et al. Ultrasound-guided low-dose interscalene brachial plexus block reduced the incidence of hemidiaphragmatic paresis. Reg Anesth Pain Med 2009;34:498–502.
[24] Mariano ER, Ilfeld BM, Cheng GS, et al. Feasibility of ultrasound-guided peripheral nerve block catheters for pain control on pediatric medical missions in developing countries. Paediatr Anaesth 2008;18:598–601.
[25] Suresh S, Chan VW. Ultrasound guided transversus abdominis plane block in infants, children and adolescents: a simple procedural guidance for their performance. Paediatr Anaesth 2009;19(1):296–9.
[26] McDonnell JG, O'Donnell B, Curley G, et al. The analgesic efficacy of transversus abdominis plane block after abdominal surgery: a prospective randomized controlled trial. Anesth Analg 2007;104(1):193–7.
[27] Visoiu M, Boretsky KR, Goyal G, et al. Postoperative analgesia via transversus abdominis plane (TAP) catheter for small weight children - our initial experience. Paediatr Anaesth 2012;22:281–4.
[28] Taylor L, Birmingham P, Yerkes E, et al. Children with spinal dysraphism: transversus abdominis plane (TAP) catheters to the rescue! Paediatr Anaesth 2010;20:951–4.
[29] Pak T, Mickelson J, Yerkes E, et al. Transverse abdominis plane block: a new approach to the management of secondary hyperalgesia following major abdominal surgery. Paediatr Anaesth 2009;19(1):54–6.
[30] Fredrickson M, Seal P, Houghton J. Early experience with the transversus abdominis plane block in children. Paediatr Anaesth 2008;18:891–2.
[31] Casati A, Baciarello M, Di Cianni S, et al. Effects of ultrasound guidance on the minimum effective anaesthetic volume required to block the femoral nerve. Br J Anaesth 2007;98: 823–7.

[32] Johnson CM. Continuous femoral nerve blockade for analgesia in children with femoral fractures. Anaesth Intensive Care 1994;22:281–3.
[33] Oberndorfer U, Marhofer P, Bosenberg A, et al. Ultrasonographic guidance for sciatic and femoral nerve blocks in children. Br J Anaesth 2007;98:797–801.
[34] Simion C, Suresh S. Lower extremity peripheral nerve blocks in children. Tech Reg Anesth Pain Manag 2007;11:222–8.
[35] Chelly JE, Greger J, Casati A, et al. Continuous lateral sciatic blocks for acute postoperative pain management after major ankle and foot surgery. Foot Ankle Int 2002;23:749–52.
[36] Dadure C, Bringuier S, Nicolas F, et al. Continuous epidural block versus continuous popliteal nerve block for postoperative pain relief after major podiatric surgery in children: a prospective comparative randomized study. Anesth Analg 2006;102:744–9.
[37] van Geffen GJ, Scheuer M, Muller A, et al. Ultrasound-guided bilateral continuous sciatic nerve blocks with stimulating catheters for postoperative pain relief after bilateral lower limb amputations. Anaesthesia 2006;61:1204–7.
[38] van Geffen GJ, Gielen M. Ultrasound-guided subgluteal sciatic nerve blocks with stimulating catheters in children: a descriptive study. Anesth Analg 2006;103:328–33.
[39] Van Geffen GJ, Pirotte T, Gielen MJ, et al. Ultrasound-guided proximal and distal sciatic nerve blocks in children. J Clin Anesth 2010;22:241–5.
[40] Van Geffen GJ, Bruhn J, Gielen M. Ultrasound-guided continuous sciatic nerve blocks in two children with venous malformations in the lower limb. Can J Anaesth 2007;54:952–3.
[41] Tsui BC, Ozelsel TJ. Ultrasound-guided anterior sciatic nerve block using a longitudinal approach: "expanding the view." Reg Anesth Pain Med 2008;33:275–6.
[42] Schwemmer U, Markus CK, Greim CA, et al. Sonographic imaging of the sciatic nerve and its division in the popliteal fossa in children. Paediatr Anaesth 2004;14:1005–8.
[43] Vas L. Continuous sciatic block for leg and foot surgery in 160 children. Paediatr Anaesth 2005;15:971–8.

Advances in Anesthesia 30 (2012) 75–96

ADVANCES IN ANESTHESIA

Anesthetic Considerations for Robotic Surgery in the Steep Trendelenburg Position

Alain F. Kalmar, MD, PhD[a,*], Andre M. De Wolf, MD[b], Jan F.A. Hendrickx, MD, PhD[c]

[a]Department of Anesthesiology, University of Groningen, University Medical Center Groningen, Hanzeplein 1, Groningen 9700 RB, The Netherlands; [b]Department of Anesthesiology, Feinberg School of Medicine, Northwestern University, 251 East Huron Street, F5-704, Chicago, IL 60611-2908, USA; [c]Department of Anesthesiology/CCM, OLV Hospital, Moorselbaan 164, Aalst 9300, Belgium

Keywords

• Robotic surgery • Trendelenburg • Prostatectomy • Anesthesiology

Key Points

- Because of the excellent results, it can be predicted that an increasing number of patients will undergo robot-assisted procedures with CO_2 pneumoperitoneum (PP) and steep Trendelenburg position. Fortunately, the human body has a remarkable yet incompletely understood capacity to withstand the effects of a CO_2 PP and steep Trendelenburg position during general anesthesia.
- Although individual responses vary and should be monitored, effects on most organs are modest and should not be an obstacle to providing optimal surgical exposure during robot-assisted prostatectomy, cystectomy, or hysterectomy. Pre-existing intracranial pathology (mass lesions and edema) needs to be excluded because it is currently the most significant absolute contraindication.
- Painstaking attention to positioning is of overriding importance. Continual awareness of the primary importance of coronary and cerebral perfusion pressures (CPPs), rather than the more common attention to mean arterial pressure (MAP), is fundamental to safeguard cardiac and cerebral perfusion.
- The interpretation of MAP needs to take the effects of height differences and site of pressure measurement into account. Further experience and study will refine the perioperative management, in particular with regard to ventilation strategies, fluid management, and postoperative analgesia.

*Corresponding author. *E-mail address*: Alain@Kalmar.be

0737-6146/12/$ – see front matter
http://dx.doi.org/10.1016/j.aan.2012.07.003

INTRODUCTION

An increasing number of surgical procedures are becoming robot assisted to optimize surgical precision, minimize incisional trauma and postoperative scarring, hasten postoperative recovery, and minimize postoperative pain. During robot-assisted surgery on the uterus, bladder, or prostate, optimal surgical exposure requires the application of a CO_2 PP with a very steep Trendelenburg position (approximately 40°). The challenges that these conditions present to anesthesiologists are reviewed.

The largest procedural and perioperative experience exists with prostatectomy, and this procedure is the focus of this review, but the concepts apply to other procedures as well. The purpose of this review is to share as much practical information as possible developed during the authors' experience in the care of more than 2000 patients [1], to review the effects of combined CO_2 PP and steep Trendelenburg position on different organs systems, to examine how this might affect choice of agents and techniques, and to identify areas that require further study.

PREOPERATIVE CONSIDERATION

Although no specific guidelines apply to the preoperative care of these patients, it may be important to rule out intracranial pathology, carotid or basilar artery disease, or glaucoma (vide infra). Particular attention to the cardiovascular and pulmonary systems review and to comorbidities of these organ systems is warranted due to the implications of laparoscopy and steep Trendelenberg positioning. Obesity may complicate further the positioning considerations (discussed later).

POSITIONING

To avoid having to repeat positioning several times, it is useful to standardize this process as much as possible. Positioning is vital to both the safety of anesthetic care and to the conduct of surgery and thus justifies the additional time and effort it often requires. Although variations in technique or equipment exist between institutions, the concepts that are presented should be widely applicable.

To prevent patients from sliding cephalad, shoulder braces are used in the authors' practice. Concern for injury to the brachial plexus has led many practices to avoid use of shoulder braces. Although a nonsliding mattress has been recommended instead of shoulder braces, this does not suffice, in the authors' experience, to prevent patients from sliding with this degree of Trendelenburg positioning [2]. The shoulders are shielded from shoulder braces with a semisoft, thick custom-made headrest (Figs. 1 and 2). The head rests against that part of the pillow that gives away slightly between both braces in an attempt to evenly distribute the body weight across the shoulders, the part of he neck that makes contact with the head rest (the spinous processes of C7 and T1), and the head of the patient (Fig. 3). Excessive pressure on the head may strain the cervical spine, whereas excessive caudad pressure on the shoulders can injure the brachial plexus [3]. The brace holders have to be placed sufficiently medial to prevent

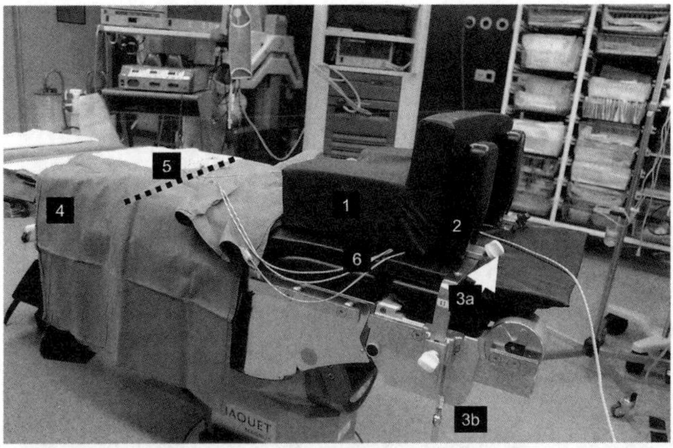

Fig. 1. Initial preparation. [1] The head is supported by a thick, soft headrest made of material that does not slide on the underlying mattress. [2] The pillow protects the shoulders from direct contact with the shoulder braces. [3a] The braces are placed sufficiently medial to prevent the head from sliding in between the two braces (also see Fig. 4); [3b] Extralong screws facilitate fixation to the side rails of the operating table. [4] The draw sheet is placed low enough so it can hold the entire hand. [5] The perineum has to align perfectly with the end of the operating table. [6] ECG cables should be placed underneath the pillow to avoid them from making skin contact because Trendelenburg increases the pressure.

the patient from sliding in-between the braces. To facilitate fixation of the braces to the side rails of the table, the authors have found extralong screws useful.

The draw sheet underneath the patient is placed low enough (before positioning the patient on the table) to ensure the arms and hands can be tucked within the sheath. To avoid direct contact or pressure of arms and hands against the leg holders, additional padding may be needed. Careful elbow padding is essential, with the thumbs in the anatomically neutral position (thumbs to the ceiling) while avoiding constrictive pressure on the arms from the drapes. When the arms are secured to the body with drapes, sliding of the patient after head-down positioning may cause a tourniquet effect, which can cause severe rhabdomyolysis and compartment syndrome, especially during lengthy procedures in obese patients [4]. Extensions have to be available for patients whose arms do not fit comfortably on the table, and the fact that there is not access to the arms during the procedure must be considered during the anesthetic planning.

INITIAL POSITIONING

First and foremost, the perineum must align with the end of the operating table that remains after removal of the bottom portion when the legs are placed in the leg holders. If a patient is too cephalad, the robot is not able to wheel-in sufficiently close to the surgical field between the patient's legs, especially if the patient slides up a few more centimeters on assuming the Trendelenburg position

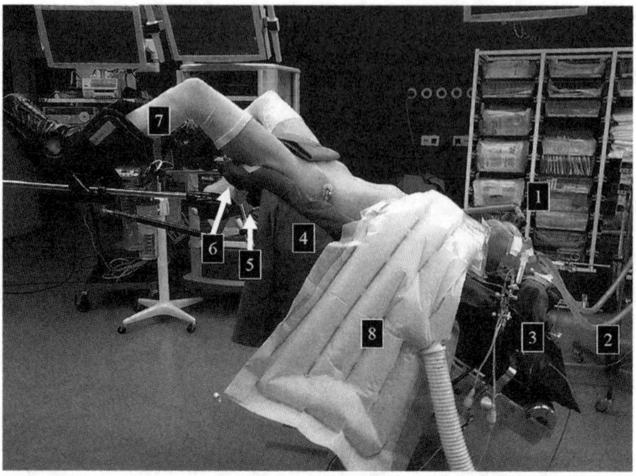

Fig. 2. The patient installed. [1] The bar of the ether screen is positioned only a few centimeters above the face to shield the face from robotic arms; a towel still needs to be placed on the face. Note absence of nasogastric tube. [2] Condensed water in the tubing could flow into the endotracheal tube if the head would be positioned lower. [3] Because the transducer is placed at the ear canal, the displayed arterial pressure will overestimate the arterial pressure at the level of the heart. [4] The circumferential pressure by the drapes around the arms should not be excessive. [5] The perineum has to perfectly align with the end of the table. [6] The draw sheet has been positioned sufficiently low so it can contain and protect the hands. [7] Both the choice of leg-holders and positioning itself are important to avoid lower leg compartment syndrome. [8] Forced warm air heating.

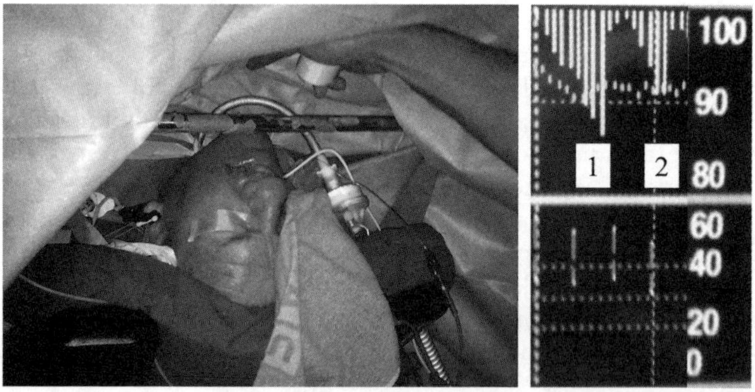

Fig. 3. Endobronchial intubation on assuming head-down tilt. Patient with the trachea intubated with an armored endotracheal tube via a preexisting tracheostomy. Little place is available to manage the airway after placing the patient in head-down tilt due to the bar of the ether screen that helps protect the face against excursions of the robotic arm. Initial endobronchial intubation [1] was recognized and the tube pulled back but reoccurred after placing the patient in Trendelenburg position [2]. (*Data from* Cassorla L, Lee JW. Patient positioning and anesthesia. In: Miller RD, Eriksson LI, Fleisher LA, et al., eds. Miller's Anesthesia. Philadelphia: Churchill Livingstone; 2009.)

(see Fig. 2). If a patient is too caudad, the pelvis may rotate, causing strain on the lumbar spine.

The choice of leg holders and positioning of the legs are important. During the bulk of the procedure, the legs have the lowest perfusion pressure because they are at the highest point relative to the heart. The authors have observed a single patient who suffered a bilateral calf compartment syndrome requiring bilateral fasciotomies, which was believed caused by a poor choice of leg holders, possibly combined with poor positioning of the legs. Enhanced attention to properly fitting and padded leg holders has been associated with no similar events since then.

ECG cables should not be positioned between the pillow and the patient's shoulders or head to avoid skin injury, and ECG pads should be applied where no direct pressure is expected.

POSTINDUCTION

No clear recommendation can be made with regard to placing a nasogastric or orogastric tube. Although some investigators argue it may prevent leakage from oral and gastric contents into the eyes during the head-down position, other investigators argue it may promote spillage by rendering the sphincters insufficient. The risk of aspiration is believed low because (1) the increased intra-abdominal pressure causes changes of the lower esophageal sphincter that allow maintenance of the pressure gradient across the gastroesophageal junction [5] and (2) the head-down position should help prevent any regurgitated fluid from entering the lower airway [6].

The Trendelenburg position and gravity cause any saliva to drip down onto the face of the patient and the towels. Because this occasionally can be pronounced, one of the authors (JFAH) prophylactically administers atropine or glycopyrrolate.

The horizontal bar of the ether screen is applied 2 cm to 3 cm above the patient's nose in an effort to allow the robotic arms to move as freely as possible (see Fig. 2). This minimum distance between the tip of the nose and the bar needs to be respected to avoid injury to the face (see Fig. 3), even after securely locking the bar into the holder on the side rails of the table. Additional padding should be applied between the nose and the bar, covering the patient's entire face. The bar and padding serves to protect the face from the robotic arms' movements and instruments that may be used above the face of the patient. The face is invisible and difficult to recognize or discern from other structures by the surgical team once the sterile drapes have covered the entire patient.

Securing the endotracheal tube is especially important, because the horizontal bar impedes further access to the airway, and the weight of breathing circuit hoses must be supported in a manner such that they do not promote the patient becoming inadvertently extubated (personal experience [JFAH]) at the beginning of the OLV Robotic Surgery Institute [1] program). After institution of the steep Trendelenburg position, cephalad migration of the carina relative to the vocal cords causes a shortening of the trachea of 0.4 ± 0.2

cm, which may result in unintentional endobronchial intubation. This may initially remain unnoticed because an increase in ventilatory pressures is anticipated, and thus confirmation of the tracheal tube positioning is recommended after patient repositioning [7,8]. In one of the authors' patients with a tracheostomy, initial endobrochial intubation of the armored tube in the supine position was recognized, the endotracheal tube was pulled back, and saturation improved, only to worsen on assuming the Trendelenburg position. It was initially suspected the CO_2 PP and Trendelenburg position were causing the desaturation, but fiberoptic bronchoscopy confirmed the tube had again migrated endobronchially (Fig. 4). Because positioning alone does not affect oxygenation in most patients (discussed later), endobronchial intubation should be suspected when desaturation occurs on assuming the Trendelenburg position.

All cables and connections (ECG cables, blood pressure cuff tubing, and so forth) need to be long enough and provide enough slack to prevent traction or impingement when a patient is placed head-down. To ensure easy intravenous access after the patient is positioned head down, an additional extension to the intravenous line can be useful. Drapes should be secured low enough relative to the surgical field so no traction is exerted after placing the patient head down. A forced air-warming blanket is applied to the upper body as a routine, but the Trendelenburg position does not require special perioperative thermal precautions or management [9].

Just before positioning the robotic arms in-between a patient's legs, the patient is brought in the full steep Trendelenburg position. This may often require the legs to be extended at the hips, with particular care taken not to overstretch the

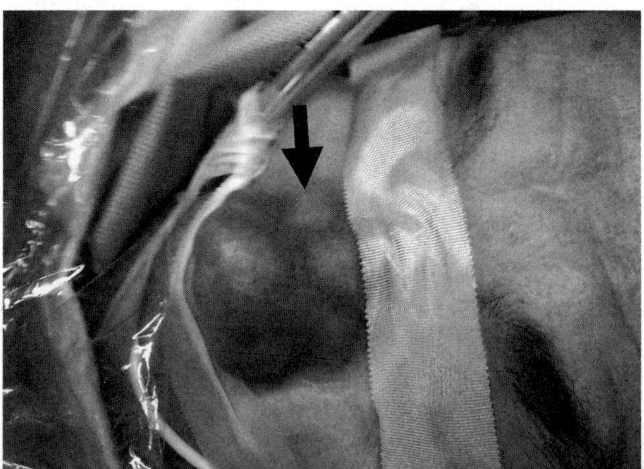

Fig. 4. Nasal injury. The bar of the ether screen has impinged (*arrow*) on the bridge of the nose. The ether screen needs to be securely fixed and the face needs to be protected. Intermittent direct inspection may be useful.

hips. It is important to remember the legs are down when the supine position is resumed much later, because this may worsen the hypotension often seen on resuming the supine position from decreased preload.

After the instruments of the robotic arms have been placed inside the patient's abdomen, the remote control of the table should be secured so it cannot inadvertently be manipulated–the consequences might be dire.

Provisions for effective communication should be established, because the noise from cooling the bulky equipment as well as the distance between the surgical field and surgeon's console makes communication difficult at times. The authors' robot has been equipped with microphones and loudspeakers.

Blood collection devices used to estimate blood loss should be placed well in sight of the anesthesiologist. Although seemingly stating the obvious, the equipment is bulky, and the room tends to become crowded.

EFFECTS ON ORGAN SYSTEMS

Hemodynamics

Hemodynamic changes during the different stages of the procedure with a 45° head-down tilt and an intra-abdominal pressure of 11 mm Hg to 12 mm Hg are presented in Fig. 5 [10]. There was no effect on cardiac performance, and filling

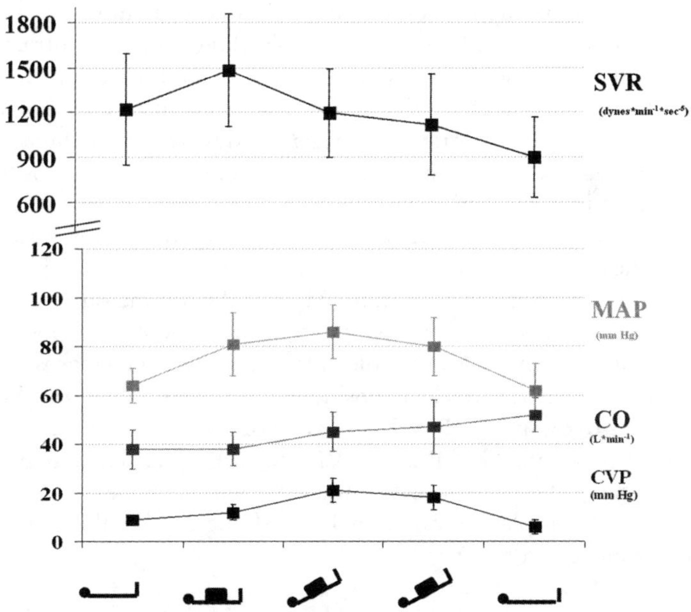

Fig. 5. Hemodynamic changes throughout the procedure. Different stages are presented in the X axis (symbols are self-explanatory). CO, cardiac output. (*Data from* Lestar M, Gunnarsson L, Lagerstrand L, et al. Hemodynamic perturbations during robot-assisted laparoscopic radical prostatectomy in 45° Trendelenburg position. Anesth Analg 2011;113(5):1069–75.)

pressures that had increased 2-fold to 3-fold normalized immediately after surgery.

Parameters of cardiac function as assessed by transesophageal echocardiography remained unchanged. Because cardiac output remains preserved during the procedure, alterations in MAP are caused by reciprocal changes in systemic vascular resistance (SVR). These blood pressure changes are most pronounced after applying the CO_2 PP (increased SVR, presumably due to direct mechanical compression of the abdominal arterial vasculature as well as neurohumoral factors [11–13]) and on resuming the supine position (decreased SVR with increased cardiac output). The latter may occasionally be pronounced; hypotension at that time can be attenuated or treated by slowly resuming the supine position, by ensuring the legs are not in the downward position, or by administering a judicious amount of phenylephrine. A constant mixed venous O_2 concentration indicates O_2 supply/demand of the body remains well preserved.

The rise in central venous pressure (CVP) immediately after assuming the steep Trendelenburg can occasionally be pronounced (>40 cm H_2O) but gradually lessens. These high filling pressures reflect the increased intrathoracic pressure from the weight of the abdominal contents on the diaphragm, rather than being indicative of hemodynamic deterioration. The intracavitary filling pressures do rise, but the transmural pressures in the right atrium and right ventricle seem largely unaffected because the right atrium and right ventricle do not enlarge on echocardiographic examination [10]. Consequently, the (very) high CVP as such does not imply a need to avoid fluids–to the contrary, a high CVP may actually mask hypovolemia [14,15]. Monitoring for trends over time is, therefore, particularly important, combined with careful monitoring of blood loss. Venous return seems well preserved during the combined CO_2 PP and Trendelenburg position because early filling flow velocity across the mitral valve is increased by 25% [10].

Nondependent areas of the body may be most at risk of hypoperfusion. When considering the coronary perfusion pressure, it is important to consider the position of the pressure transducers used for MAP and CVP measurements. When placing a patient in the steep Trendelenburg position, the vertical position of the external ear canal relative to the middle of the right atrium increases by approximately 20 cm. If the transducer is positioned at the ear canal, the MAP (and CVP as well) is overestimated by 20 cm H_2O or 14.7 mm Hg. CPP, however, does not change because MAP and CVP increase by an equivalent amount. Therefore, placing the transducers at the ear canal allows easy calculation of the CPP, but risks displaying deceivingly satisfying MAP values for the heart and nondependent body parts.

Gas exchange

Although the individual effects of a CO_2 PP and moderate degrees of head-up or head-down tilt separately on pulmonary gas exchange have been well described [6,16], until recently few data existed on their combined effects on lung function.

Induction of anesthesia decreases the functional residual capacity and thus the alveolocapillary membrane surface across which gas exchanges occur. Even though a CO_2 PP and steep Trendelenburg position are expected to worsen atelectasis and further reduce the functional residual capacity of the lung, a study the authors performed showed that venous admixture did not change, and changes in dead space ventilation were modest (which was also indicated by the absence partial pressure of end-expired CO_2 [P_ECO_2]/$Pa{CO_2}$ changes) (Fig. 6) [17].

The approximately 50% dead-space ventilation (including apparatus dead space) throughout the procedure is almost identical to the 51% reported during general anesthesia [18]. The 10% venous admixture the authors found is of the order of magnitude that can be expected after induction of anesthesia [18]. Half of this venous admixture is caused by atelectasis resulting in absolute shunt, and the other half by dispersion of the distribution of perfusion to alveoli with low ventilation-perfusion ratios resulting in ventilation-perfusion mismatch.

Other investigators have found that increasing intra-abdominal pressure to 14 mm Hg with more moderate degrees of head-down (−20°) did not significantly modify physiologic dead space or venous admixture [16,19,20]. Even more surprisingly, Andersson and colleagues [21,22] found that, despite increasing atelectasis, CO_2 PP transiently reduces venous admixture, thereby increasing arterial oxygenation, a finding corroborated by other studies [23,24]. Why CO_2 PP increases arterial oxygenation despite increasing atelectatic lung area on CT by 66% (range, 11%–170%) has not been elucidated. Andersson and colleagues [21] suggest that the CO_2 PP might improve ventilation-

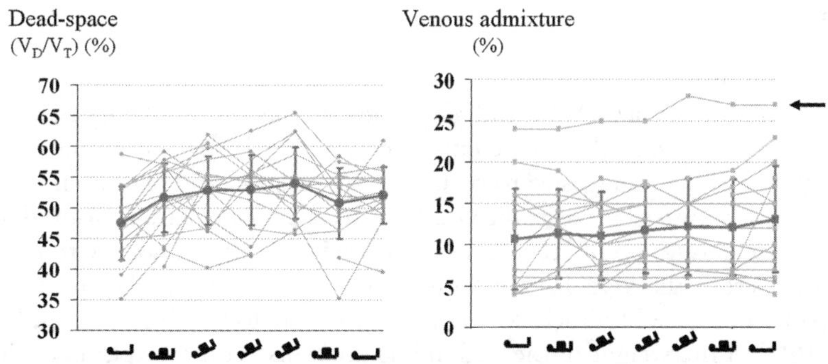

Fig. 6. Effects on dead-space ventilation and venous admixture. Dead-space ventilation (expressed as dead-space/tidal volume [V_D/V_T] [%]) and venous admixture. Thick lines with bars represent average and SD, respectively. Changes in dead-space ventilation are modest, and venous admixture did not change. Even in a patient with significant preexisting venous admixture (*arrow*), oxygenation did not worsen significantly. (*Data from* Schrijvers D, Mottrie A, Traen K, et al. Pulmonary gas exchange is well preserved during robot assisted surgery in steep Trendelenburg position. Acta Anaesthesiol Belg 2009;60(4):229–33.)

perfusion matching because the increased intra-abdominal pressure transmitted to the thorax could decrease perfusion in those areas where shunting was prevalent before PP. This theory is supported by a decreased dispersion of blood flow after induction of PP, which indicates better matching. Increased pulmonary capillary P_{CO_2} also enhances hypoxic pulmonary vasoconstriction.

It remains remarkable that lung function does not become more impaired under these nonphysiologic conditions. Even in a patient with a 25% venous admixture after induction of anesthesia (Fig. 6), venous admixture did not worsen after applying a PP or steep Trendelenburg position [17]. Although these results are reassuring and average gas exchange is unaltered, it should remain appreciated that there is considerable interindividual variability (Fig. 6) [25,26]. At some stage during the procedure, an individual patient may, therefore, benefit from a higher F_{IO_2}, an alveolar recruitment maneuver with or without the application of positive end-expiratory pressure (PEEP) (eg, after resuming the supine position), or an increase in minute ventilation. It is imperative to carefully monitor the arterial saturation with pulse oximetry and the end-expired CO_2 concentration and, if warranted, use arterial blood gas analysis to assess the alveolar-arterial O_2 and CO_2 gradients. Still, the intraoperative effects of CO_2 PP and steep Trendelenburg, in particular, on dead-space ventilation and venous admixture are small and should not be an obstacle to providing optimal surgical exposure by providing steep Trendelenburg position.

Whether or not to apply PEEP is somewhat unclear. Reasons not to apply PEEP are (1) the inconsistency with which low levels of PEEP have been proved effective [27–29]; (2) oxygenation is already improved by the CO_2 PP; (3) intrathoracic pressures increase further; and (4) venous drainage of the central nervous system (CNS) may be impeded. Although Valenza and colleagues [15] suggest PEEP be used, the value of recruitment maneuvers is being investigated.

Lung mechanics

The combination of a CO_2 PP and Trendelenburg alters ventilatory mechanics, mainly by decreasing thoracic compliance (Fig. 7) [14,15]. Although several strategies have been suggested to curb increases in peak and plateau inspiratory pressures, it is important to realize that (1) these pressures are measured at the mouthpiece and (2) do not reflect the pressure in the alveoli nor the transmural pressure across the alveoli. The bulk of the increase in airway pressures is caused by decreased thoracic wall compliance (due to pressure exerted by the CO_2 PP and the weight of the abdominal contents on the diaphragm) due to the head-down position–any changes in lung compliance are comparatively small. This is fortunate, because it implies that overdistention of the alveoli is not occurring despite the elevation seen in airway pressures. Alveoli are distended by an increase in transmural pressure across the alveolar (or lung) wall (transmural pressure = alveolar pressure − intrapleural pressure). Because the pressures in the pleural space and the alveoli are increased to the same degree (due to the decrease in thoracic wall compliance), lung transmural pressure and

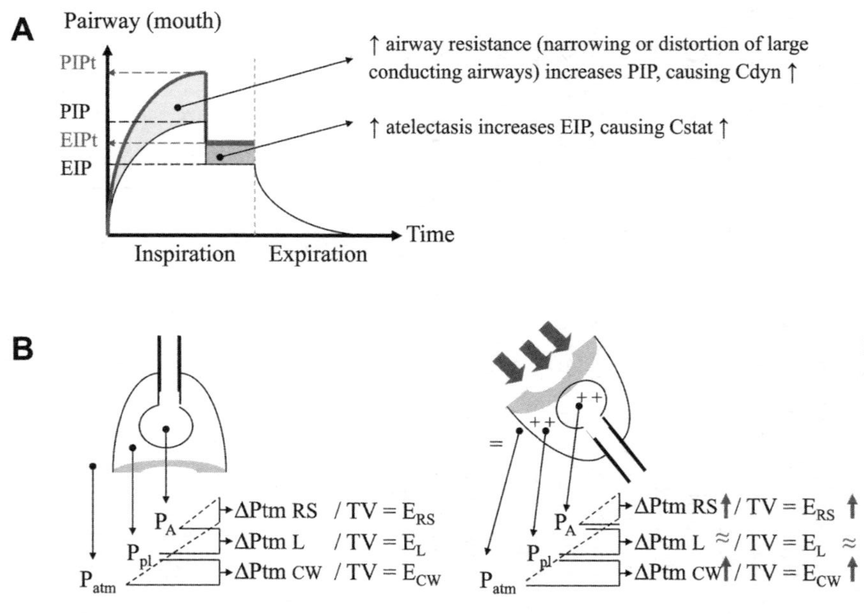

Fig. 7. The rise of airway pressure measured at the mouth is a poor descriptor of the mechanical derangement occurring during CO_2 PP. (*A*) When using controlled mechanical ventilation, applying CO_2 PP and head-down tilt causes a rise in both the peak inspiratory pressure (PIP) (because the large airways become distorted or narrowed) and the end-inspiratory (or plateau) pressure (EIP) (due to atelectasis), resulting in decreased dynamic (Cdyn) and static (Cstat) compliance. (*B*) These high airway pressures, however, do not pose the patient at risk of barotrauma or volutrauma because the transmural pulmonary pressure is unchanged. The increased airway pressure is the result of increased chest wall elastance (= E_{CW}) (or decreased chest wall compliance – elastance is the reciprocal of compliance) due to the pressure of the CO_2 PP and the weight of abdominal contents. The increased airway pressure (paw) is not the result of increased lung elastance (= E_L). Elastance of the entire respiratory system (RS) consisting of the sum of lungs (L) and the chest wall (CW) is increased ($E_{RS} = E_L + E_{CW}$), causing Paw to rise. Transmural gradients (ΔPtm) are calculated from the alveolar pressure (P_A), intrapleural pressure (P_{pl}), and atmospheric pressure (P_{atm}). Elastance is the ratio of the tidal volume (TV) and the ΔPtm under consideration. (*Data from* Valenza F, Chevallard G, Fossali T, et al. Management of mechanical ventilation during laparoscopic surgery. Best Pract Res Clin Anaesthesiol 2010;24(2):227–41.)

thus alveolar dimensions have not changed. Therefore, the high airway pressures as such do not have to be treated–ventilation can be continued with normal tidal volumes, and the airway pressures can often be followed without undue concern. Note that the decreased chest wall elastance is also contributory to the misleading high CVP values (discussed previously) (Fig. 8).

Still, absorption and elimination of exogenous CO_2 require additional ventilation, up to 30% to maintain normocapnia [16]. Any increase in end-expired CO_2 larger than 25% or occurring later than 30 minutes after the beginning of the CO_2 PP should suggest CO_2 subcutaneous emphysema [6].

To attenuate the peak airway pressure, during controlled mechanical ventilation, tidal volume may be decreased and respiratory rate and the duration of the inspiratory phase increased (eg, inspiratory-expiratory ratio from 1:2 to 1:1). Pressure-controlled ventilation may limit the inspiratory pressures, but the tidal volume becomes dependent on the constantly changing resistive and compliance characteristics of the lungs–careful titration relative to the end-expired CO_2 is mandatory if this approach is chosen.

The pressure-controlled volume guarantee or analogous ventilation mode available on some anesthesia machines uses software that adjusts the inspiratory flow pattern to deliver the required tidal volume with the lowest airway pressure possible. Somewhat surprisingly, this mode does not automatically manipulate the inspiratory-expiratory ratio, which is an important tool to attenuate airway pressures by allowing more inspiratory time.

No ventilation mode has been proved superior [30–32]. Although different ventilatory modes have been proposed, it is more important to understand

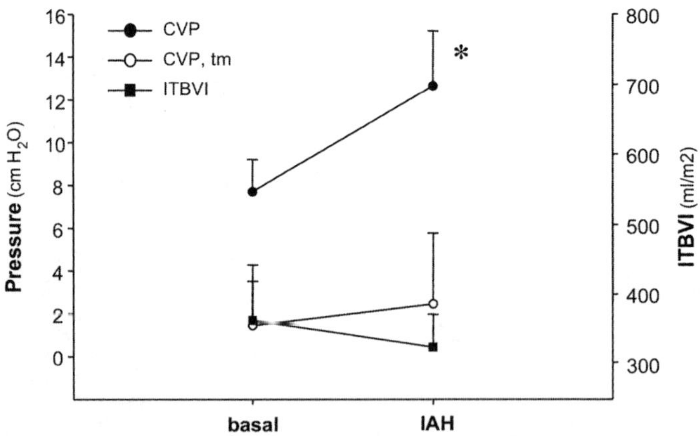

Fig. 8. The role of chest wall derangement on high CVP values during CO_2 PP. During intra-abdominal hypertension (IAH), CVP significantly rises whereas transmural pressure (CVP, tm) or intrathoracic blood volume (ITBVI) do not, underlying the role of chest wall derangement on artifactually and potentially misleading high CVP values during CO_2 PP. (*Data from* Valenza F, Chevallard G, Fossali T, et al. Management of mechanical ventilation during laparoscopic surgery. Best Pract Res Clin Anaesthesiol 2010;24(2):227–41.)

why the pressures increase and that the pressures at the mouthpiece do not reflect alveolar nor transmural lung pressure.

If maintaining isocapnia proves a challenge despite adjustments to the ventilator, $PACO_2$ can be allowed to rise (permissive hypercapnia), which is generally well tolerated for the duration of the procedure. This may be an option particularly with excessive resorption of CO_2 from the retroperitoneum. Although CO_2 resorption from within the peritoneum is modest, CO_2 that finds its way outside the peritoneum via the surgical site (the prostate is located outside the peritoneum) or in-between the peritoneum and the other structures making up the abdominal wall may lead to excessive exogenous CO_2 absorption that can strain the CO_2 removal capacity of the lungs (vide infra). Finally, the intraperitoneal abdominal CO_2 pressure may have to be decreased or temporarily released to briefly hyperventilate the patient and bring $Paco_2$ down to acceptable levels (exceptionally rare). Because the increase in $Paco_2$ depends on the intra-abdominal pressure, reducing it may help decrease $Paco_2$ [33].

CNS

Patients generally tolerate even prolonged episodes of CO_2 PP well: after several tens of thousands of patients have undergone a robot-assisted prostatectomy, the authors are aware of no reports of focal or global neurologic deficits. Why do patients tolerate even prolonged (>6 hours) exposure to the combination of combined CO_2 PP and steep Trendelenburg position so well?

First, CNS blood flow (CBF) is autoregulated (Fig. 9). Within certain limits of perfusion pressure, CBF remains constant because the diameter of the cerebral arterioles increases as CPP decreases. If CNS perfusion behaves like a Starling resistor (see Fig. 9), CPP is the difference between MAP and either CVP or intracranial pressure (ICP), depending on which is highest. The lower threshold of autoregulation is often cited as 50 mm Hg to 60 mm Hg (although these thresholds have been challenged) [34].

The authors have found that the average CPP (calculated as MAP − CVP) after assuming the Trendelenburg position remains within the limits, between which CBF is usually considered maintained by autoregulation [35]. Later, however, during the course of the procedure, CPP may drop well below 50 mm Hg in an occasional patient (Fig. 10). Even though an effect on outcome cannot be claimed, some anesthesiologists argue this is an indication to invasively monitor MAP and CVP. The authors use this information to guide administration of phenylephrine to restore CPP above 60 mm Hg. By positioning the transducer at the level of the ear canal, CPP can be directly calculated from the mean values displayed on the monitor. The high CVP and MAP values displayed on the monitors are not indicative of a sufficient filling status and perfusion pressure of more elevated organs, respectively.

Second, CO_2 PP increases ICP. This increase is independent of arterial pH, oxygenation, or MAP; it is seen even at low (8 mm Hg) abdominal pressures and is especially pronounced in animals with baseline elevated ICP [36–38].

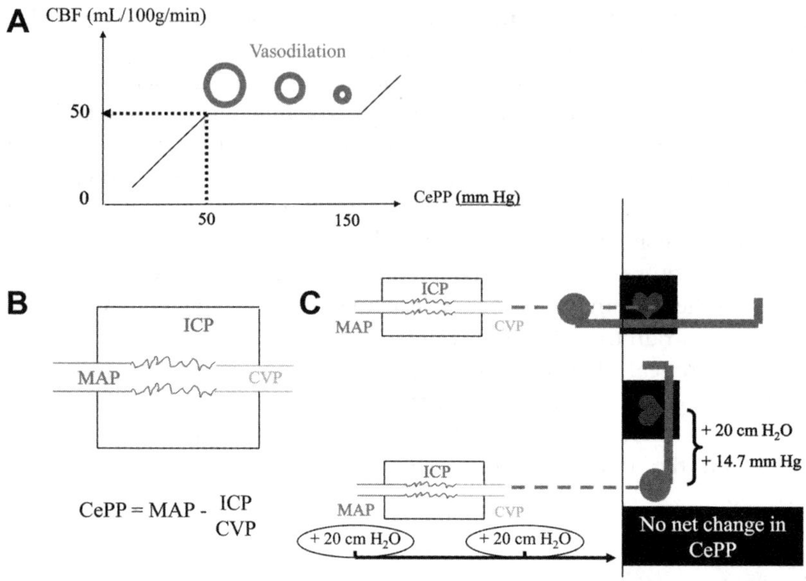

Fig. 9. Autoregulation, CPP, and positioning of pressure transducers. (*A*) Blood flow to the brain (CBF) is autoregulated within certain limits: as the cerebral perfusion pressure (CePP) decreases, cerebral vessels dilate, maintaining CBF. Below a CePP of 50 mm Hg, CBF decreases with CePP (even though the exact relationship is probably more complex, and varies between individuals). (*B*) If CNS perfusion is likened to a Starling resistor, CePP can be calculated as the difference between MAP and CVP or ICP, whichever is higher. MAP and CVP can be easily measured; CPP cannot be higher than the difference between these two (but it could be lower, if ICP is higher than CVP, although ICP is not measured). (*C*) If the pressure transducer is positioned at the ear canal, and the patient is placed head down, both MAP and CVP rise by an equal amount (eg, 20 cm H_2O or 14.7 mm Hg), resulting in no net change in CePP. The high MAP in and by itself may give a false sense of adequate perfusion pressure – the MAP at the level of the coronary arteries is 14.7 mm Hg lower.

Trendelenburg position worsens the increase in ICP during insufflation, but reverse Trendelenburg does not eliminate it [36]. The exact mechanism by which intraabdominal pressure affects ICP has not been elucidated, but it is probably multifactorial [39]. The Monro-Kellie doctrine states that the bony skull contains 3 elements: parenchymal tissue, arterial and venous blood, and cerebrospinal fluid in a dynamic equilibrium. With a rapid increase in the volume of any of these components, ICP rises. It has been proposed that increased intraabdominal and intrathoracic pressure as well as impaired cerebrospinal fluid absorption during insufflation impede drainage of the lumbar venous plexus and induce an increase in the vascular compartment of the sacral space, causing the rise in ICP [36,40]. Additionally, hypercarbia is known to cause cerebral vasodilation, which results in an increased ICP. If ICP does not increase, an increased transmural vascular pressure might render the intracerebral vessels prone to rupture.

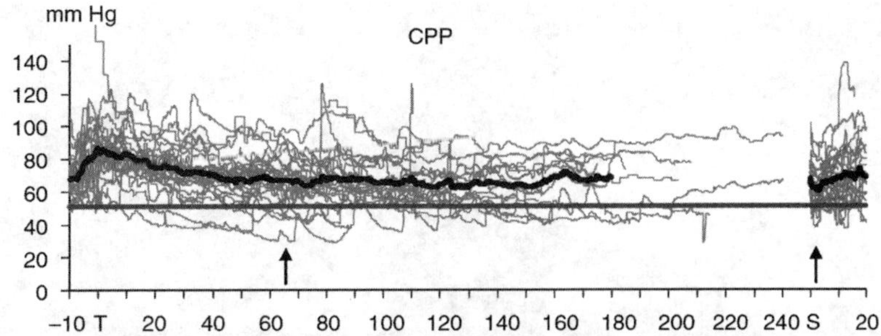

Fig. 10. Average CPP calculated as MAP – CVP remained within autoregulatory limits after assuming the Trendelenburg position. Later, however, during the course of procedure, CPP may drop well below 50 mm Hg in an occasional patient (see curves below red line). Even though an effect on outcome cannot be claimed, some anesthesiologists argue this is an indication to invasively monitor MAP and CVP. (*Data from* Kalmar AF, Foubert L, Hendrickx JF, et al. Influence of steep Trendelenburg position and CO2 pneumoperitoneum on cardiovascular, cerebrovascular, and respiratory homeostasis during robotic prostatectomy. Br J Anaesth 2010;104(4):433–9.)

Third, there are important surrogate outcome variables that indicate the brain tolerates the CO_2 PP and steep Trendelenburg position well. Using near-infrared spectrometry, the authors have found regional brain oxygenation well preserved (Fig. 11). During initiation of the surgery program at the authors' institution, a CT scan of the brain of one patient before and immediately after the procedure (<15 minutes) revealed no abnormalities (Fig. 12). No evidence was found of increased resistance to CBF, indicating that any cerebral edema that might have developed would be unlikely to affect cerebral perfusion [41]. In addition, the authors' preliminary findings of optic nerve sheath diameter

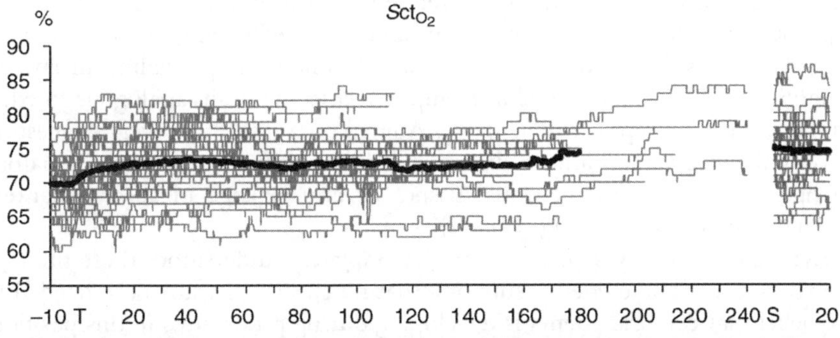

Fig. 11. Effects of CO_2 PP and head-down positioning on near-infrared spectroscopy. In 31 patients, regional cerebral tissue saturation ($Scto_2$) increased on average from 70% to 73%, after assuming the Trendelenburg position, and further increased to 74%, after resuming the supine position. (*Data from* Kalmar AF, Foubert L, Hendrickx JF, et al. Influence of steep Trendelenburg position and CO2 pneumoperitoneum on cardiovascular, cerebrovascular, and respiratory homeostasis during robotic prostatectomy. Br J Anaesth 2010;104(4):433–9.)

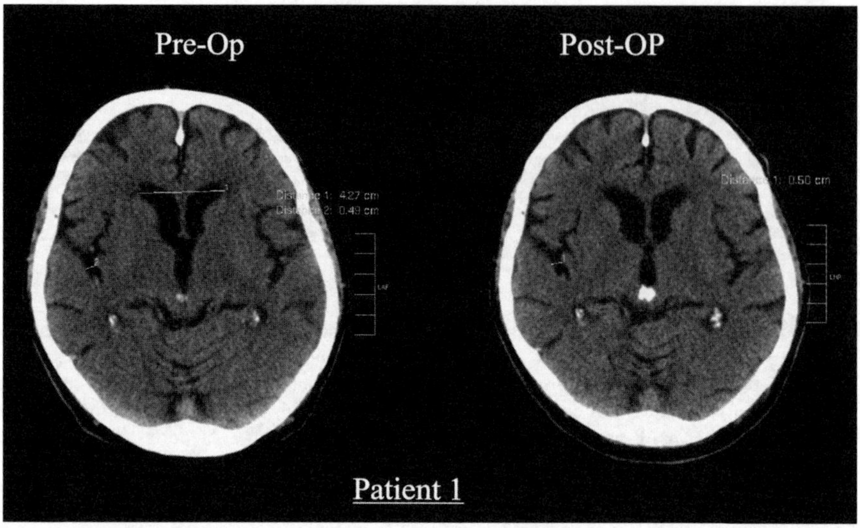

Fig. 12. CT scan of the brain. During initiation of the surgery program at the authors' institution, a CT scan of the brain of 3 patients before and immediately after the procedure (<15 minutes) revealed no abnormalities.

measurements (a well-documented indicator of increased ICP in the acute trauma setting) are reassuring.

Fourth, even though facial edema may develop, this is by no means indicative of intracerebral fluid kinetics. The blood-brain barrier helps prevent the development of interstitial edema in the CNS despite the increase of the hydrostatic pressure in the cerebral blood vessels. The composition of intracerebral capillaries (the blood-brain barrier) is entirely different from that of the extracranial capillaries (Fig. 13). Useful information can be gleaned from space research: the head-down position is used to simulate the conditions prevailing in space—weightlessness causes a fluid shift from the feet to the brain analogous to what happens during steep Trendelenburg. Animal data (rabbits) reveal congestion of only the pial vessels after 8 days of head-down tilt without any edematous changes of the cerebral neuronal tissues or any leakage of special markers through the vessel walls (Fig. 14) [42].

Even though many aspects remain incompletely understood, these findings are reassuring. The evidence supports that no special measures are needed in the belief that cerebral edema is developing during procedures in this position. There are limits, however, and common sense needs to guide clinical judgment in certain circumstances (eg, a 75-year-old male patient with a preoperative diagnosed space-occupying lesion in the medullary region should not undergo robotic radical cystectomy) [43]. The authors expect that any condition that may disturb the blood-brain barrier (such as brain tumors) carries unknown risks which the available data do not allow fully understanding or anticipating.

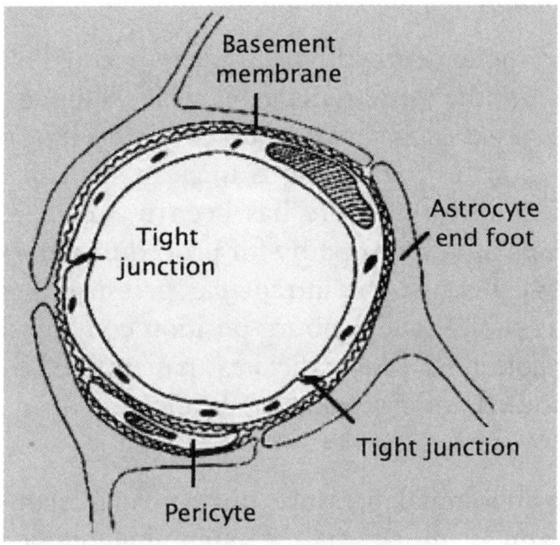

Fig. 13. Histology of the blood-brain barrier. The gaps between endothelial cells of the CNS are sealed by tight junctions. Pericytes and endothelial cells are completely encapsulated by basement membrane. Astrocytic end-feet envelop approximately 99% of all the vasculature.

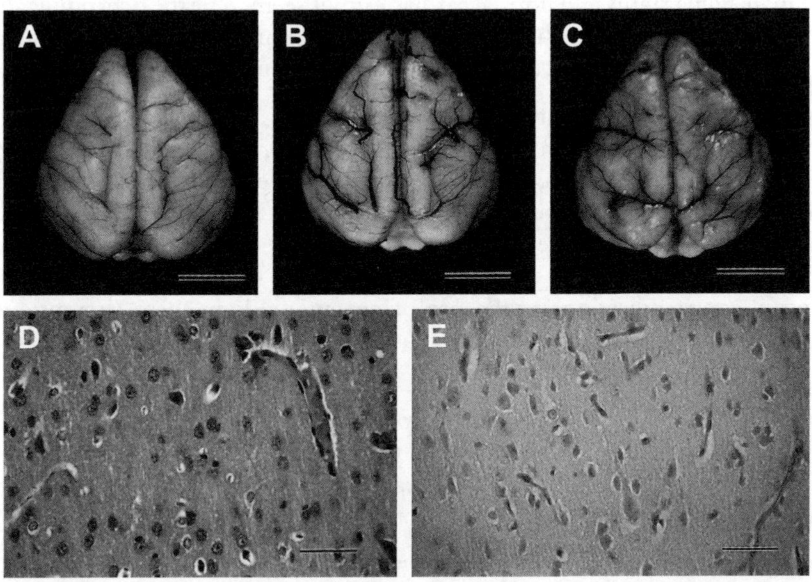

Fig. 14. Histopathology of the blood-brain barrier after 8 days of head-down tilt. Animal data (rabbits) reveal congestion of the pial vessels only after sustained (*A* = controll, *B* = after 2 days, *C* = after 8 days) head-down tilt , without any ... neuronal tissues (light microscopical findings of the cortex in the frontal lobe excised from the 8-day head down tilt rabbit and stained with hematoxylin and eosin, *D*) or leakage of the special markers through the vessel walls (immunohistochemical staining of the cortex in the frontal lobe excised from the 8-day head down tilt rabbit, *E*). (*Data from* Shimoyama R, Miyata H, Ohama E, et al. Does edema formation occur in the rabbit brain exposed to head-down tilt? Jpn J Physiol 2000;50(1):141–7.)

Posterior ischemic optic neuropathy has been reported after minimally invasive prostatectomy, but the cause remains unclear. Although anamnesis should reveal ocular pathology during the preoperative interview, its value in preventing ocular complications in this setting is unclear. Even in patients with glaucoma or other ocular diseases, there has been no reported increased risk of perioperative ischemic optic neuropathy for procedures in the prone or Trendelenburg position [44]. Because the intraocular pressure increases, on average, 13 mm Hg by the end of Trendelenburg position compared with preinduction values, however, common sense dictates patients with glaucoma should continue their scheduled antiglaucoma medication.

Renal

Elevations of intra-abdominal pressure during laparoscopic procedures may lead to oliguria or anuria in mammals. Despite this, previous research has not been able to confirm an associated kidney injury and none could be found in a recent study where rats were exposed to a CO_2 PP of up to 4 hours: urine output was reduced but NGAL expression, a sensitive marker for renal injury, was not increased [45]. The authors are aware of no data on the renal effect of Trendelenburg position nor on its combined use with a CO_2 PP. Maintaining an adequate filling status and normal cardiac output seem to be the overriding goals to preserve renal function; under these conditions, urinary output is unlikely to be a predictor of postoperative renal dysfunction [46,47].

Choice of anesthetic agents

No particular drug regimen has been shown superior with regard to meaningful outcome in this population, and either a total intravenous technique or inhaled anesthetic technique can be used. Nitrous oxide is not specifically contraindicated–it does not interfere with surgical exposure [48] and it may promote a rapid emergence. Although there is always a risk of venous air embolism, it is not a contraindication for the use of nitrous oxide in these circumstances and none has been reported during robot-assisted laparoscopies.

Fluid management

Whether colloids should be preferred to crystalloids is speculative, but because facial edema resulting from head-down tilt in volunteers is caused primarily by elevated capillary pressures and decreased plasma colloid osmotic pressures [49], it may be wise to avoid overzealous administration of crystalloids.

Emergence and postoperative care

Postoperative agitation has been observed but remains poorly quantified, and the contribution of the CO_2 PP and Trendelenburg position is uncertain. Despite indirect evidence to the contrary, it has prompted some anesthesiologists to speculate that cerebral edema might be present and ventilate patient postoperatively arbitrarily for 1 hour. Arguing that an awake patient is the best neuromonitor, other investigators (JFAH) prefer to extubate the patients immediately postoperatively. The cause of postoperative agitation is probably multifactorial, and intensive postoperative analgesia and the administration of an anticholinergic drug to attenuate bladder spasm and the discomfort of the presence of a Foley catheter seems to have lessened its incidence in the authors' experience. Transversus abdominis plane blocks placed after induction of anesthesia may help provide additional postoperative analgesia. Readers may infer from the absence of references in this section that more questions remain than have been answered.

It is imperative to ensure that the airway can be maintained after extubation. Although facial and scleral edema is an important physical sign that can alert clinicians to the presence of airway edema, significant edema of pharyngeal tissue may not be accompanied by visible external signs. Laryngeal soft tissue edema may be assessed by performing a cuff leak test: gas should be able to flow past the endotracheal tube after deflating the cuff when a pressure of 15 cm H_2O is applied. Another option is to have the patient breathe spontaneously and to occlude the proximal end of the endotracheal tube after cuff deflation–the patient should ideally then be able to breathe around the tube. Postextubation respiratory distress may require reintubation and subsequent ventilation in an ICU [3]. The authors recommend that if the cuff leak test fails, patients should remain intubated until the edema has subsided. Other indications for (brief) postoperative ventilation may include excessive blood loss or excessive subcutaneous emphysema.

Furosemide may be prescribed by a urologist in an attempt to prevent blood clot formation in the urinary tract. Although the evidence to substantiate this practice is scant or nonexistent, its side effects are well documented: hypokalemia, hyperglycemia, hypovolemia, and loss of urinary output as an indicator of organ perfusion. If administered, appropriate fluid administration to compensate for excessive urine production and electrolyte loss should be considered.

Contraindications

The major contraindication is intracranial pathology associated with intracranial hypertension or disruption of the blood-brain barrier. In patients suffering from glaucoma, it is probably wise to ensure the ocular pressure has been well treated.

SUMMARY

Because of the excellent results, it can be predicted that an increasing number of patients will undergo robot-assisted procedures with CO_2 PP and steep Trendelenburg position. Fortunately, the human body has a remarkable yet incompletely understood capacity to withstand the effects of a CO_2 PP and steep Trendelenburg position during general anesthesia. Although individual responses vary and should be monitored, effects on most organs are modest and should not be an obstacle to providing optimal surgical exposure during robot-assisted prostatectomy, cystectomy, or hysterectomy. Pre-existing intracranial pathology (mass lesions and edema) needs to be excluded because it is currently the most significant absolute contraindication. Painstaking attention to positioning is of overriding importance. Continual awareness of the primary importance of coronary and CPPs, rather than the more common attention to

MAP, is fundamental to safeguard cardiac and cerebral perfusion. The interpretation of MAP needs to take the effects of height differences and site of pressure measurement into account. Further experience and study will refine the perioperative management, in particular with regard to ventilation strategies, fluid management, and postoperative analgesia.

References

[1] Available at: http://www.olvroboticsurgeryinstitute.eu/olv.
[2] Cassorla L, Lee JW. Patient positioning and anesthesia. In: Ronald D. Miller, editor. Anesthesia. New York, London: Churchill Livingstone; 2009. p. 1819–87.
[3] Phong SV, Koh LK. Anaesthesia for robotic-assisted radical prostatectomy: considerations for laparoscopy in the Trendelenburg position. Anaesth Intensive Care 2007;35(2):281–5.
[4] Deras P, Amraoui J, Boutin C, et al. Rhabdomyolysis and compartment syndrome of two forearms after robotic assisted prolonged surgery. Ann Fr Anesth Reanim 2010;29(4):301–3 [in French].
[5] Jones MJ, Mitchell RW, Hindocha N. Effect of increased intra-abdominal pressure during laparoscopy on the lower esophageal sphincter. Anesth Analg 1989;68(1):63–5.
[6] Joris J. Anesthesia for laparoscopic surgery. In: Ronald D. Miller, editor. Anesthesia. New York, London: Churchill Livingstone; 2009. p. 2185–202.
[7] Burton A, Steinbrook RA. Precipitous decrease in oxygen saturation during laparoscopic surgery. Anesth Analg 1993;76(5):1177–8.
[8] Morimura N, Inoue K, Miwa T. Chest roentgenogram demonstrates cephalad movement of the carina during laparoscopic cholecystectomy. Anesthesiology 1994;81(5):1301–2.
[9] Nakajima Y, Mizobe T, Matsukawa T, et al. Thermoregulatory response to intraoperative head-down tilt. Anesth Analg 2002;94(1):221–6, table of contents.
[10] Lestar M, Gunnarsson L, Lagerstrand L, et al. Hemodynamic perturbations during robot-assisted laparoscopic radical prostatectomy in 45 degrees Trendelenburg position. Anesth Analg 2011;113(5):1069–75.
[11] Joris JL, Noirot DP, Legrand MJ, et al. Hemodynamic changes during laparoscopic cholecystectomy. Anesth Analg 1993;76(5):1067–71.
[12] Sharma KC, Brandstetter RD, Brensilver JM, et al. Cardiopulmonary physiology and pathophysiology as a consequence of laparoscopic surgery. Chest 1996;110(3):810–5.
[13] Viinamki O, Punnonen R. Vasopressin release during laparoscopy: role of increased intra-abdominal pressure. Lancet 1982;1(8264):175–6.
[14] Valenza F, Chevallard G, Porro GA, et al. Static and dynamic components of esophageal and central venous pressure during intra-abdominal hypertension. Crit Care Med 2007;35(6):1575–81.
[15] Valenza F, Chevallard G, Fossali T, et al. Management of mechanical ventilation during laparoscopic surgery. Best Pract Res Clin Anaesthesiol 2010;24(2):227–41.
[16] Tan PL, Lee TL, Tweed WA. Carbon dioxide absorption and gas exchange during pelvic laparoscopy. Can J Anaesth 1992;39(7):677–81.
[17] Schrijvers D, Mottrie A, Traen K, et al. Pulmonary gas exchange is well preserved during robot assisted surgery in steep Trendelenburg position. Acta Anaesthesiol Belg 2009;60(4):229–33.
[18] Lumb A. Nunn's applied respiratory physiology. 6th edition. Butterworth-Heinemann; 2005.
[19] Bures E, Fusciardi J, Lanquetot H, et al. Ventilatory effects of laparoscopic cholecystectomy. Acta Anaesthesiol Scand 1996;40(5):566–73.
[20] Odeberg-Wernerman S, Sollevi A. Cardiopulmonary aspects of laparoscopic surgery. Curr Opin Anaesthesiol 1996;9:529–35.
[21] Andersson LE, Baath M, Thorne A, et al. Effect of carbon dioxide pneumoperitoneum on development of atelectasis during anesthesia, examined by spiral computed tomography. Anesthesiology 2005;102(2):293–9.

[22] Andersson L, Lagerstrand L, Thorne A, et al. Effect of CO2 pneumoperitoneum on ventilation-perfusion relationships during laparoscopic cholecystectomy. Acta Anaesthesiol Scand 2002;46(5):552–60.
[23] Kelman GR, Swapp GH, Smith I, et al. Caridac output and arterial blood-gas tension during laparoscopy. Br J Anaesth 1972;44(11):1155–62.
[24] Odeberg S, Sollevi A. Pneumoperitoneum for laparoscopic surgery does not increase venous admixture. Eur J Anaesthesiol 1995;12(6):541–8.
[25] McMahon AJ, Baxter JN, Kenny G, et al. Ventilatory and blood gas changes during laparoscopic and open cholecystectomy. Br J Surg 1993;80(10):1252–4.
[26] Wahba RW, Mamazza J. Ventilatory requirements during laparoscopic cholecystectomy. Can J Anaesth 1993;40(3):206–10.
[27] Bruells CS, Rossaint R. Physiology of gas exchange during anaesthesia. Eur J Anaesthesiol 2011;28(8):570–9.
[28] Hedenstierna G, Edmark L. The effects of anesthesia and muscle paralysis on the respiratory system. In: Pinsky M, Brochard L, Mancebo J, et al, editors. Applied physiology in intensive care medicine. Dordrecht (The Netherlands), Heidelberg (Germany), London, New York: Springer-Verlag; 2009. p. 390.
[29] Pelosi P, Ravagnan I, Giurati G, et al. Positive end-expiratory pressure improves respiratory function in obese but not in normal subjects during anesthesia and paralysis. Anesthesiology 1999;91(5):1221–31.
[30] De Baerdemaeker LE, Van der Herten C, Gillardin JM, et al. Comparison of volume-controlled and pressure-controlled ventilation during laparoscopic gastric banding in morbidly obese patients. Obes Surg 2008;18(6):680–5.
[31] Balick-Weber CC, Nicolas P, Hedreville-Montout M, et al. Respiratory and haemodynamic effects of volume-controlled vs pressure-controlled ventilation during laparoscopy: a cross-over study with echocardiographic assessment. Br J Anaesth 2007;99(3):429–35.
[32] Choi EM, Na S, Choi SH, et al. Comparison of volume-controlled and pressure-controlled ventilation in steep Trendelenburg position for robot-assisted laparoscopic radical prostatectomy. J Clin Anesth 2011;23(3):183–8.
[33] Lister DR, Rudston-Brown B, Warriner CB, et al. Carbon dioxide absorption is not linearly related to intraperitoneal carbon dioxide insufflation pressure in pigs. Anesthesiology 1994;80(1):129–36.
[34] Ng JL, Chan MT, Gelb AW. Perioperative stroke in noncardiac, nonneurosurgical surgery. Anesthesiology 2011;115(4):879–90.
[35] Kalmar AF, Foubert L, Hendrickx JF, et al. Influence of steep Trendelenburg position and CO2 pneumoperitoneum on cardiovascular, cerebrovascular, and respiratory homeostasis during robotic prostatectomy. Br J Anaesth 2010;104(4):433–9.
[36] Halverson A, Buchanan R, Jacobs L, et al. Evaluation of mechanism of increased intracranial pressure with insufflation. Surg Endosc 1998;12(3):266–9.
[37] Josephs LG, Este-McDonald JR, Birkett DH, et al. Diagnostic laparoscopy increases intracranial pressure. J Trauma 1994;36(6):815–8 [discussion: 818–9].
[38] Rosenthal RJ, Hiatt JR, Phillips EH, et al. Intracranial pressure. Effects of pneumoperitoneum in a large-animal model. Surg Endosc 1997;11(4):376–80.
[39] Grabowski JE, Talamini MA. Physiological effects of pneumoperitoneum. J Gastrointest Surg 2009;13(5):1009–16.
[40] Este-McDonald JR, Josephs LG, Birkett DH, et al. Changes in intracranial pressure associated with apneumic retractors. Arch Surg 1995;130(4):362–5 [discussion: 365–6].
[41] Kalmar AF, Dewaele F, Foubert L, et al. Cerebral haemodynamic physiology during steep Trendelenburg position and CO2 pneumoperitoneum. Br J Anaesth 2012;108(3):478–84.
[42] Shimoyama R, Miyata H, Ohama E, et al. Does edema formation occur in the rabbit brain exposed to head-down tilt? Jpn J Physiol 2000;50(1):141–7.
[43] Pandey R, Garg R, Darlong V, et al. Unpredicted neurological complications after robotic laparoscopic radical cystectomy and ileal conduit formation in steep trendelenburg position: two case reports. Acta Anaesthesiol Belg 2010;61(3):163–6.

[44] Awad H, Santilli S, Ohr M, et al. The effects of steep trendelenburg positioning on intraocular pressure during robotic radical prostatectomy. Anesth Analg 2009;109(2):473–8.
[45] de Barros RF, Miranda ML, de Mattos AC, et al. Kidney safety during surgical pneumoperitoneum: an experimental study in rats. Surg Endosc 2012. Available at: http://dx.doi.org/10.1007/s00464-012-2322-4.
[46] Knos GB, Berry AJ, Isaacson IJ, et al. Intraoperative urinary output and postoperative blood urea nitrogen and creatinine levels in patients undergoing aortic reconstructive surgery. J Clin Anesth 1989;1(3):181–5.
[47] Alpert RA, Roizen MF, Hamilton WK, et al. Intraoperative urinary output does not predict postoperative renal function in patients undergoing abdominal aortic revascularization. Surgery 1984;95(6):707–11.
[48] Brodsky JB, Lemmens HJ, Collins JS, et al. Nitrous oxide and laparoscopic bariatric surgery. Obes Surg 2005;15(4):494–6.
[49] Parazynski SE, Hargens AR, Tucker B, et al. Transcapillary fluid shifts in tissues of the head and neck during and after simulated microgravity. J Appl Physiol 1991;71(6):2469–75.

Advances in Anesthesia 30 (2012) 97–129

ADVANCES IN ANESTHESIA

Modern and Evolving Understanding of Cerebral Perfusion and Autoregulation

Nathaniel H. Greene, MD[a], Lorri A. Lee, MD[a,b,*]

[a]Department of Anesthesiology and Pain Medicine, University of Washington, Seattle, WA 98195-6540, USA; [b]Department of Neurological Surgery, University of Washington, Seattle, WA 98195-6540, USA

Keywords

• Cerebral perfusion • Cerebral blood flow • Autoregulation
• Lower limit of autoregulation • Cerebrovascular reactivity • Cerebral ischemia
• Beach chair position • Cerebral perfusion pressure

Key Points

- Significant changes in anesthetic management for optimizing cerebral perfusion have occurred over the past 5 to 10 years. Perhaps the most important of these changes has been a reinterpretation of older autoregulation studies that have resulted in raising the lower limit of autoregulation to approximately 70 mm Hg to 80 mm Hg, and not the previously used 60 mm Hg.
- Tremendous variability in the lower limits of autoregulation exists among individuals. Using a percentage reduction below baseline blood pressure as a lower limit may result in better optimization of cerebral perfusion than using absolute blood pressure values.
- Other changes in practice for the general anesthesiologist include correcting blood pressure for height differences between the site of blood pressure measurement and the brain, particularly in the sitting position, to account for the hydrostatic gradient. Rare cases of severe brain damage have been reported that may be related to hypoperfusion in the beach chair position.
- Multiple physiologic and drug interactions that affect cerebral perfusion occur during every general anesthetic, and understanding the best way to optimize cerebral blood flow may potentially improve outcomes. Newer research on flow-metabolism coupling points to regional control of cerebral blood flow by the neurovascular unit, with glial cells playing a central role.

Disclosures: Dr Greene and Dr Lee report no financial disclosures.

*Corresponding author. Department of Anesthesiology and Pain Medicine, University of Washington, 1959 Northeast Pacific Street, Box 356540–BB 1469, Seattle, WA 98195-6540. *E-mail address:* lorlee@uw.edu

0737-6146/12/$ – see front matter
http://dx.doi.org/10.1016/j.aan.2012.08.003

INTRODUCTION

Defining the parameters that affect cerebral perfusion and understanding the pathophysiologic conditions that result in a supply and demand mismatch is of paramount concern for anesthesiologists. Stroke is one of the most devastating perioperative complications, and can occur with an incidence of 0.1% to 1.0% in patients undergoing noncardiac, non-neurological procedures, using national database statistics [1]. It is difficult to estimate what percentage of these perioperative strokes are related to embolic phenomena versus hypoperfusion, but hypoperfusion was strongly implicated as a causative factor in the multicenter randomized controlled trial Perioperative Ischemic Evaluation Study (POISE), in which patients receiving perioperative beta blockade had a twofold increased risk of stroke compared with patients who received placebo [2]. Retrospective single-institution studies have also found a significant relationship between perioperative stroke and intraoperative hypotension [3]. In contrast, a recent review of the literature noted that hypoperfusion was causative in only 6.6% of the 301 strokes identified [4]; yet, several studies have suggested that hypoperfusion may exacerbate the effect of microemboli. The indirect evidence suggests that "low" mean arterial pressure (MAP) may increase the risk of a perioperative stroke in certain high-risk individuals, but defining "low" for all patients and all procedures is problematic.

The goal of this article was to enhance the reader's understanding about factors that affect cerebral blood flow (CBF), and to reexamine some misperceptions from earlier clinical studies on cerebral autoregulation and their impact on clinical practice. Rarer neurologic complications, such as ischemic optic neuropathy related to the prone and steep Trendelenburg positions, and severe brain damage in the sitting position, that highlight the potentially deleterious impact of patient position on cerebral perfusion are also discussed.

FUNDAMENTALS OF CBF

Humans have long been interested in cerebral perfusion and the brain as far back as 2800 BC, but it was not until the mid-1900s that the first techniques to measure CBF were developed by Kety and Schmidt (Fig. 1) [5–7]. We now have at least 18 different methods for measuring CBF, with newer tools of analysis, such as functional magnetic resonance imaging and positron emission computed tomography, that can demonstrate 3-dimensional images of CBF to a resolution of less than 1 cm [6]. Widespread use of these newer techniques should improve our understanding of cerebral perfusion to better guide our clinical practice.

Inherent to understanding perfusion of the brain is first understanding the immense metabolic requirement of the brain. The brain makes up only 2% of the body weight, but receives as much as 15% to 20% of the cardiac output, approximately 50 to 60 mL/100 g brain tissue/min, or 750 to 1000 mL/min in an adult. It consumes as much as 20% of the total oxygen requirement at resting conditions at 3.3 mL/100 g brain tissue/min [5,6]. Of the oxygen used, 40% is devoted to what is known as basal metabolism: homeostasis of

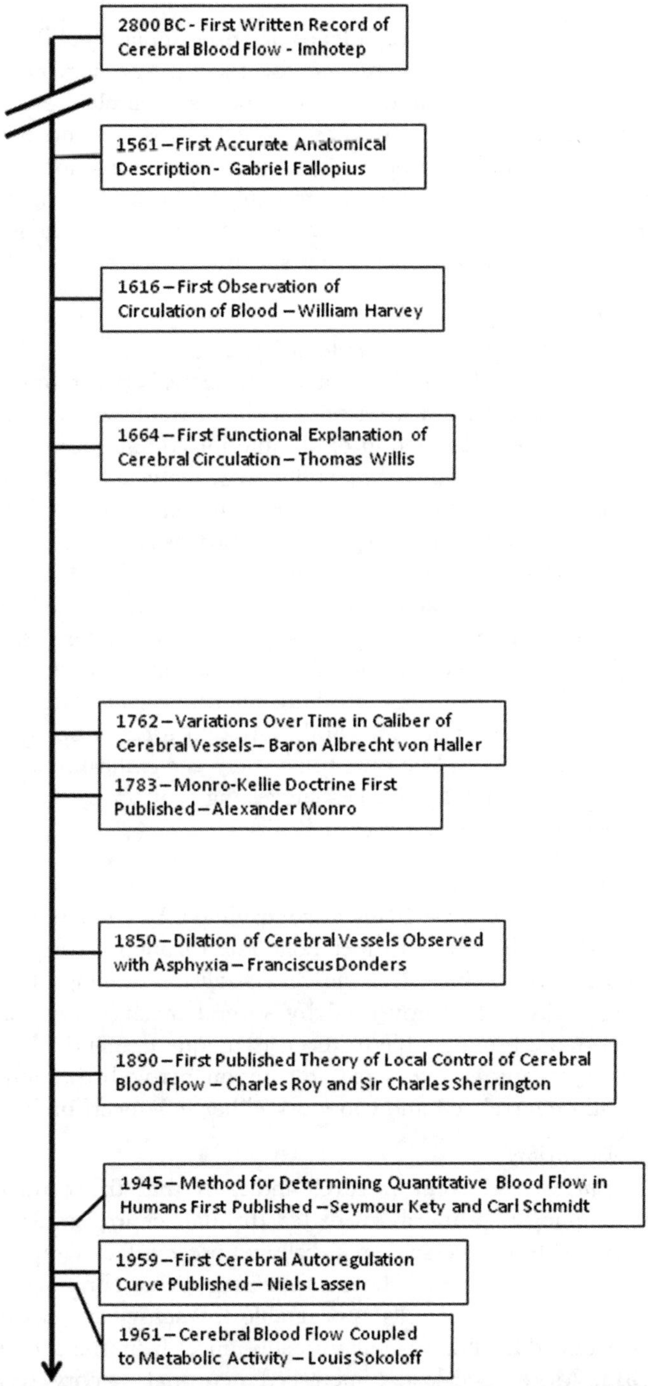

Fig. 1. Timeline of important milestones in the history of cerebral perfusion research. *Data from* Refs. [5–7].

the neuronal networks, providing adenosine triphosphate (ATP) to maintain ion gradients, and providing substrate for the central nervous system to communicate (ie, neurotransmitters, polypeptides, complex proteins). The other 60% is necessary for what is known as activation or functional metabolism: the energy required to support electrophysiologic function and to allow the neurons of the brain to communicate [5,6]. Because of its high metabolic activity and relatively low energy storage capacity, the brain is especially vulnerable to interruption of oxygen and substrate delivery.

Circle of Willis

In its most simple description, the circle of Willis is a continuous arterial circle that forms at the base of the brain by interconnections between branches of the left and right internal carotid arteries and the vertebrobasilar system. This circle is made because of formation of an anterior communicating artery that connects the left and right internal carotid systems between both anterior cerebral arteries, and the formation of posterior communicating arteries bilaterally that connect the carotid systems to the vertebrobasilar system between the middle cerebral arteries and the posterior cerebral arteries. Willis seemed to put it best after he made his anatomic discovery when he wrote "if by chance one or two should be stopt, there might easily be found another passage instead of them" [7]. The circle receives blood from 4 distinct sources that directly come from branches of the aorta with both internal carotid arteries being fed via the common carotid artery and both vertebral arteries being fed via the subclavian arteries. It should be noted that there is significant variance in the human population, with some studies suggesting that fewer than half of the population possess a complete circle of Willis.

Control of CBF

There are several different mechanisms controlling CBF. The brain has adapted the ability to match CBF with metabolic rate through a variety of physiologic mechanisms, better known as flow-metabolism coupling. This coupling can occur regionally and is governed by several mechanisms that serve as the basis of how the brain is able to meet its unique demands. It is useful to separate these mechanisms into separate components with the understanding that they are still interrelated and can work either in concert or in opposition.

Chemical/metabolic control

The neurovascular unit. Current research indicates that the control of flow-metabolism coupling is primarily mediated through neurovascular units consisting of cerebral blood vessels, glial cells whose endfeet wrap around the vessels, and perivascular nerve fibers innervating the cerebral vessels and the glial cells (Box 1). The glial cells appear able to "sense" increased neuronal activity and release diffusible vasodilatory substances from the endfeet, thereby affecting CBF. More specifically, increased neuronal activity results in an increase in glial intracellular calcium, causing a release of ATP and glutamate [8]. ATP is involved in recruiting adjacent glial cells to respond as a unit via

Box 1: Control of CBF

Control of CBF is centered around the neurovascular unit, which consists of the following:

- Perivascular nerve fibers innervating glial cells and blood vessels
- Glial cells with endfeet that wrap around cerebral vessels
- Cerebral vessels

Diffusible substances are secreted by the nerve fibers and glial cells, which affect CBF and increase connectivity of the neurovascular unit. The vascular endothelium also contributes to control of CBF. Glutamate affects both metabolism and CBF.

propagation of calcium waves. One of the many effects of glutamate is to stimulate production of nitric oxide (NO), which is a cerebral vasodilator and thought to be involved in the regulation of flow-metabolism coupling. Glutamate also activates glial cells via metabotropic glutamate receptors with subsequent calcium signaling and arachadonic acid formation. Arachadonic acid, or its lipid derivatives, serve as vasodilatory or vasoconstrictor substances released by the glial endfeet surrounding the cerebral blood vessels. NO, K+, H+, brain metabolites, such as adenosine and lactate, and O_2 influence the direction of vascular tone [9]. K+ and H+ ions are produced by synaptic transmission, and increases in their concentrations stimulate cerebral vasodilation. Glutamate uptake by glial cells generates sodium waves that subsequently increase glucose uptake and metabolism. The increased lactate production from this metabolism is used by neurons as an energy substrate [8]. Glutamate increases connectivity of glial cells with neurons and capillaries (the neurovascular unit) as it affects both metabolism and CBF. The glial cells (astrocytes) play a vital role in local flow–metabolism coupling.

The perivascular nerve endings of cerebral vessels are also thought to be involved in flow-metabolism coupling via release of neurotransmitters, such as norepinephrine, acetylcholine, substance P, somatostatin, cholecystokinin, vasoactive intestinal peptide, calcitonin gene-related peptide, epoxyeicosatrienoic acids (EETs), and others [10]. EETs are arachidonic acid metabolites, which are potent cerebral vasodilators and are also produced by astrocytes and the vascular endothelium. The source of innervation for this cerebral microvasculature (or "intrinsic innervation") is unknown in humans, but is thought to arise from the nucleus basalis, locus coeruleus, and raphe nucleus in animals [6]. The extrinsic innervation for flow-metabolism coupling is discussed later in this article.

Carbon dioxide. CO_2, the main by-product of aerobic respiration, is a potent cerebral vasodilator and provides a very basic model of regulation by shifting blood toward more metabolically active tissues. A linear relationship exists between CBF and CO_2 tension throughout normal physiologic values of CO_2 (20–75 mm Hg), with an approximate 2% to 6% change in CBF per mm Hg CO_2 [6,11,12]. The effect of changes in CO_2 on CBF depends on the underlying vascular tone and competing demands on CBF, as there is a point of maximal vasodilation (and vasoconstriction) beyond which the vessel cannot further alter its diameter. For example, profound hypotension can greatly diminish CO_2 reactivity because the cerebral vessels are maximally vasodilated. Similarly, hypercapnia can impede autoregulation for the same reasons.

The mechanism of CO_2 reactivity is related to changes in the pH of the extracellular fluid surrounding the brain. Low-pH solutions topically applied to the brain surface cause vasodilation, whereas high-pH solutions cause vasoconstriction. CO_2, unlike H+ ions, readily diffuses across the blood brain barrier and cerebral endothelium [6]. Consequently, CO_2 changes have a relatively quick effect on CBF, but metabolic acidosis has little immediate effect on CBF. Because the cerebrospinal fluid actively eliminates bicarbonate with prolonged hyperventilation and normalizes its pH, effects on CBF typically revert to baseline within approximately 6 hours, even though the arterial partial pressure of CO_2 ($Paco_2$) may remain low. Thus, acute correction of $Paco_2$ after prolonged hyperventilation can lead to pronounced increases in CBF, which may have deleterious effects on patients with raised intracranial pressure (ICP) [6].

The change in vascular tone caused by CO_2 is partially mediated by NO, as inhibitors of NO synthase will diminish the vasodilatory response to hypercapnia. NO modulation of cerebrovascular tone occurs through combined activation of ATP-sensitive and calcium-activated potassium channels in animal studies [13]. Indomethacin, an inhibitor of cyclooxygenase and prostaglandin formation, will partially inhibit the vasodilatory response to increasing CO_2 concentrations in humans. Experimental studies in animals show that application of prostaglandin E2 (PGE2) after indomethacin administration will restore the cerebrovascular reactivity to baseline, as PGE2 is thought to stimulate production of endothelial NO synthase [14]. Studying these mechanisms at this level of complexity has been difficult, as they have been shown to differ depending on the animal studied.

Pao_2, arterial O_2 content, and rheology. Oxygen (O_2), also exhibits regulatory capacity, as CBF increases when O_2 levels start to drop below 60 mm Hg in humans [15]. Early studies in normocapnic rats showed that CBF significantly increased at Pao_2 levels as high as 85 mm Hg, but that marked increases up to 500% of baseline CBF occurred within 1 to 2 minutes at a Pao_2 of 25 mm Hg [16]. NO synthase inhibitors given to humans partially blocked this response, suggesting that it is partially regulated by NO [17]. Chemoreceptors in the periphery and neuraxis, and hyperpolarization of vascular smooth muscle via ATP-dependent potassium channels, may also contribute to hypoxia-induced vasodilation [6].

Hypoxemia increases CBF to a greater degree than hemodilution, at the same arterial O_2 content (CaO_2) [18]. Hemodilution has been well documented in animal and human studies to increase CBF and raise the lower limit of autoregulation (LLA) [18,19]. Both the decreased viscosity with improved rheology, and reduced CaO_2 are responsible for the increase in CBF with hemodilution, based on studies in animals [20]. Although NO is involved in cerebral vasodilation with reduced CaO_2 from hypoxemia, it does not appear to contribute to increased CBF with reduced viscosity [18].

Temperature. Temperature-induced changes in CBF are a reflection of changes in the cerebral metabolic rate of O_2 ($CMRO_2$). As a patient's temperature drops, there is a corresponding drop in $CMRO_2$ from both basal and functional metabolism, estimated to be approximately 7% for each 1°C between 37°C and 27°C [5]. Isoelectric electroencephalogram (EEG) occurs at temperatures of 18 to 20°C. Pharmacologic suppression, which only affects functional metabolism, is synergistic with hypothermic suppression until EEG silence. At that point, $CMRO_2$ can be reduced only by further drops in temperature [6]. Numerous smaller studies have documented the improved survival and outcomes using mild to moderate hypothermia in traumatic brain injury (TBI) and other pathologic states, and the deleterious effects of hyperthermia. Larger randomized controlled trials of hypothermia in traumatic brain injury and during clipping of cerebral aneursyms have not demonstrated a beneficial effect for all patients [21,22]. Hypothermia seems to be neuroprotective during vulnerable periods of cerebral ischemia in successfully resuscitated cardiac arrest patients [23].

One of the few studies in humans with hyperthermia and controlled ventilation showed that increasing temperatures to 41.8°C with propofol anesthesia decreased O_2 extraction by 1.6-fold and increased middle cerebral artery blood flow velocity by 1.5-fold, with partial impairment of autoregulation [24]. It was suggested that the decreased O_2 extraction was a consequence of a similar increase in CBF, and that $CMRO_2$ may actually have been stable. In animals, $CMRO_2$ increases up to 42°C, and then falls to baseline values or lower at 43°C, presumably because of metabolic dysfunction and impending cell death. In contrast to anesthetized subjects with controlled ventilation, research in awake, spontaneously ventilating humans and animals revealed that CBF decreased with hyperthermia, largely because of an associated increase in ventilation and reduced $Paco_2$ (Box 2) [25].

Neurogenic control

In addition to the extensive network of perivascular nerve endings associated with the neurovascular unit discussed previously, neurogenic control of CBF

Box 2: Physiologic parameters affecting CBF

- Carbon dioxide
- Pao_2/arterial O_2 content
- Temperature
- Viscosity/rheology
- Sympathetic/Parasympathetic stimulation
- Myogenic control/autoregulation

Anemia increases CBF by its effect on viscosity/rheology and arterial O_2 content.

is also mediated via sympathetic (adrenergic), parasympathetic (cholinergic), and sensory neurons that innervate vessels outside of the brain tissue, sometimes referred to as the "extrinsic innervation" [26]. The extrinsic system of neurogenic control of CBF is thought to exert its most pronounced effect on the large cerebral arteries. The sympathetic nervous system associated with the superior cervical ganglion influences vascular tone to maintain blood pressure below the upper limit of autoregulation [27]. Sympathetic stimulation can alter the autoregulatory curve and push it to the right, possibly providing a protective effect during periods of acute hypertension [28,29]. Intense stimulation of the sympathetic nervous system has been shown to cause a significant decrease in CBF, whereas local blockade of the sympathetic nervous system can provide a significant increase in CBF [28,30]. In a study using baboons, in which autoregulation was intact to 35% of baseline blood pressure when hypotension was drug induced, autoregulation was intact to only 65% of baseline blood pressure when hypotension was induced by controlled hemorrhage, suggesting that activation of the sympathetic nervous system during hemorrhage contributed to a higher LLA [31]. The role of lower cardiac output in this scenario was not elucidated, but numerous studies suggest that acute hypovolemia may narrow the range of autoregulatory capacity and raise the LLA via activation of the sympathetic nervous system.

The parasympathetic nervous system is associated with the sphenopalatine and otic ganglia and is more functional during disease or injury states, such as Alzheimer disease, with decreased cholinergic innervation [26]. However, both the cholinergic and adrenergic nerves are thought to be involved in exercise-induced changes in CBF and metabolism. Sensory neurons work through the trigeminal ganglion and are important for pain sensation [26]. The discovery of trigeminal neurons in mediating migraine pain via the vasodilator, calcitonin gene-related peptide (CGRP), has led to the development of triptan drugs that inhibit release of CGRP presynaptically and cause cerebral vasoconstriction.

Myogenic control/autoregulation

In the healthy resting human, CBF is kept constant over a wide range of cerebral perfusion pressures (CPP) via cerebral vasoconstriction and vasodilation. This concept is known as *autoregulation* and seems to exist in humans, as well as in other vertebrates. It is a process whereby changes in CPP cause changes in cerebrovascular resistance to maintain a constant CBF. Cerebral autoregulation protects the brain from hypoxia at low CPP, and against hyperemia, capillary leakage, and vasogenic edema at high CPP. As the cerebral vessels have limits to how wide they can dilate and how small they can constrict, there are limits to this autoregulatory capacity, and if exceeded, blood flow becomes *pressure passive* and is subject to changes in systemic blood pressure. The LLA is the CPP when there is maximal cerebral vasodilation. The upper limit of autoregulation (ULA) is the CPP where there is maximal cerebral vasoconstriction (Fig. 2). Autoregulatory ranges vary greatly among individuals and within an individual depending on other influences on vascular tone (eg, $Paco_2$, hemoglobin concentration, anesthetic agents). Older

Factors Decreasing Cerebral Blood Flow

	CBF	$CMRO_2$
Vasoactive Drugs		
Hypotensive Agents		
β Blockers	↓/0	↓/0
α2 Agonist	↓	↓/0
Nitric Oxide Donors	↓/0/↑	↓/0
Vasopressors/Inotropes/Chronotropes		
α1 Agonist	↓/0	0
Dopamine (high dose)	↓	0
Norepinephrine	↓/0	0/↑
Vasopressin	0	0
Anesthetic Drugs		
Intravenous Agents		
Barbiturates	↓↓	↓↓
Etomidate	↓↓	↓↓
Propofol	↓↓	↓↓
Benzodiazepines	↓	↓
Synthetic Opioids	0	↓/0
Volatile Agents		
Xenon	↓(Gray)/↑(White)	↓
Isoflurane (0.5 - 1 MAC)	0	↓↓
Sevoflurane (0.5 - 1 MAC)	↓/0	↓/↓↓
Desflurane (0.5 -1 MAC)	↓	↓↓
Physiologic Parameters		
$PaCO_2$ < 40 mm Hg	↓↓	0
PaO_2 >300 mm Hg	0/↓	0
Temperature < 37° C	↓	↓
Viscosity (↑)	↓	0

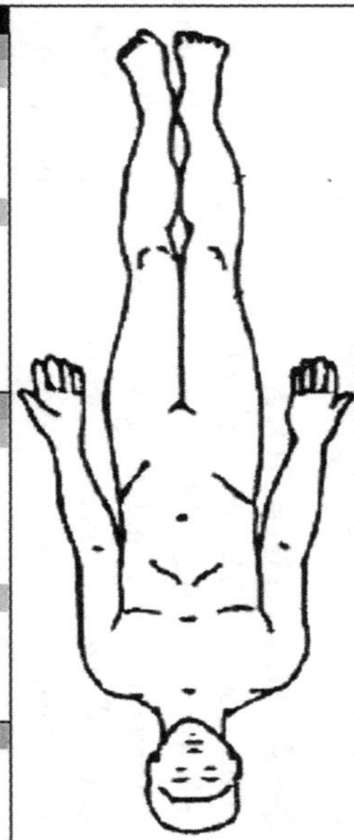

Factors Increasing Cerebral Blood Flow

	CBF	$CMRO_2$
Vasoactive Drugs		
Hypotensive Agents		
Calcium Channel Blockers	↑/0	↑/0
Nitric Oxide Donors	↓/0/↑	↓/0
Vasopressors/Inotropes/Chronotropes		
β Agonist	↑	↑
β Agonist (BBB open)	↑↑↑	↑↑↑
Dopamine (low dose)	↑↑	0
Norepinephrine (BBB open)	↑	↑
Epinephrine	↑	↑
Epinephrine (BBB open)	↑↑↑	↑↑↑
Anesthetic Drugs		
Intravenous Agents		
Ketamine	↑↑	0/↑
Ketamine (w/ other anesthetics)	↓/0	↓/0
Volatile Agents		
Nitrous Oxide	↑↑	0/↑
Isoflurane (2 MAC)	↑↑	↓↓
Sevoflurane (2 MAC)	↑↑	↓/↓↓
Desflurane (2 MAC)	↑↑	↓↓
Physiologic Parameters		
Temperature > 37° C	↑	↑
PaO_2 < 60 mm Hg	↑↑	0
$PaCO_2$ > 40 mm Hg	↑↑	0
Anemia	↑	0

*The above parameters assume that blood pressure is within the normal autoregulatory window

**It should be noted these are isolated effects, and that the effect of simultaneous factors may be additive or they may diminish or completely abolish an effect on CBF.

Fig. 2. Pharmacology of CBF. Drugs and physiologic parameters that affect CBF and autoregulation.*, **

texts have cited limits of autoregulation in healthy patients under normal physiologic conditions at a CPP of 50 mm Hg (approximate MAP of 60 mm Hg) at the LLA and 140 mm Hg (approximate MAP 150 mm Hg) at the ULA. Reinterpreting these older studies for clinical translation has led to a revision of the LLA to a MAP of 70 mm Hg in healthy adults, (see section Lower Limit of Autoregulation that follows) [6].

The process by which autoregulation occurs is unknown but is relatively slow, taking approximately 2 or more minutes for CBF to adjust to baseline values after an acute drop in MAP. Autonomic innervations of the central nervous system and NO may have contributory roles to the mechanism of autoregulation [32]. Increases in transmural pressure are known to induce an endothelium-derived factor that induces smooth muscle depolarization. This depolarization causes a conformational change in the actin-myosin complex of the smooth muscle cells within seconds and results in vasoconstriction. Recent research has detected mechanoreceptors within the smooth muscle cells themselves. Depolarization of these nonselective mechanosensitive ion channels results in an influx of Ca++ and smooth muscle constriction. Increased flow velocity exerts increased shear stress and can cause vasoconstriction independent of transmural pressure [26].

LOWER LIMIT OF AUTOREGULATION

Historical interpretation of the LLA for cerebral ischemia

The LLA commonly refers to the MAP (or CPP) on the CBF versus MAP (or CPP) autoregulatory curve in which the cerebral blood vessels are maximally dilated, and in which CBF becomes pressure passive if MAP (or CPP) is further lowered (Fig. 3). In the past, the LLA has erroneously been thought of as an absolute number for all patients. Instead, it varies among and within individuals, and depends on the state of multiple other physiologic parameters and pharmacologic agents that may influence cerebral sympathetic tone and limit the extent of autoregulatory capacity. It has received great attention because of the implications for blood pressure management under anesthesia in normal and diseased states. Because intact neurologic function cannot be assessed, even with today's best technology, under moderate to deep sedation or general anesthesia, anesthesiologists have always been interested in defining the lower limit of "safe" blood pressure whereby adequate cerebral perfusion is ensured if blood pressure is maintained above this lower limit. Although one could always keep the MAP, no lower than baseline values to ensure adequate CPP, this practice may have the unintended consequences of increased bleeding in some procedures, and could promote harmful side effects of increased blood transfusion, or other fluid or vasoactive medication administration.

Blood pressures lower than a predetermined LLA do not necessarily result in immediate and irreparable brain damage. The duration and extent of the decrease in CPP below the LLA are important, with less dramatic decreases being tolerated for longer duration. Awake healthy subjects developed symptoms of cerebral ischemia at CBF of 24 to 38 mL/100 g/min [33]. Although most studies

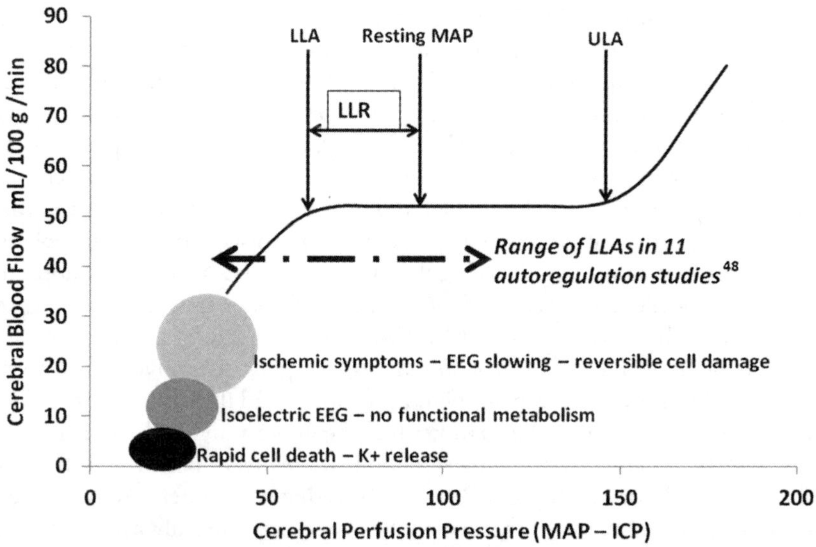

Fig. 3. Autoregulation curve. The cerebral vasculature maintains a stable CBF over a wide range of CPP (typically CPP 60–140 or MAP 70–150 mm Hg). The lower end of the autoregulatory range is the LLA, where there is maximal cerebral vasodilation. The ULA is when there is maximal cerebral vasoconstriction. The area between the baseline MAP and the LLA is known as the lower limit reserve (LLR). Symptoms and signs (EEG slowing) of cerebral ischemia occur at approximately 24 to 38 mL/100 g/min CBF and neuronal damage is still reversible. Functional metabolism ceases between 15 and 6 mL/100 g/min with an isoelectric EEG, and neurons will eventually die. Destruction of cell integrity occurs at approximately CBF <6 mL/100 g/min and rapid cell death ensues. The lower the CBF at ischemic levels, the shorter the duration allowable before irreversible neuronal damage. The dashed-dotted line represents the range of LLAs from 11 autoregulation studies in awake humans. (*Data from* Drummond JC. The lower limit of autoregulation: time to revise our thinking? Anesthesiology 1997;86(6):1431–3.)

in anesthetized humans and primates report that EEG or evoked potential changes do not occur until CBF declines to approximately 20 mL/100 g/min [34,35], preexisting neuronal injury may raise that threshold to as high as 39 mL/100 g/min [36]. Other factors that may reduce O_2 delivery, such as anemia or low PaO_2, or increase in $CMRO_2$, may raise the CBF threshold in which ischemia develops. In anesthetized primates at a CBF of 15 mL/100 g/min, functional metabolism ceases as demonstrated by an isoelectric EEG, and below 6 mL/100 g/min, cell integrity is potentially irreversibly threatened [37]. Although irreversible brain damage will not occur if a patient's MAP briefly drops below his or her LLA, keeping the MAP above the LLA should provide some margin for error, assuming other physiologic conditions are normal.

Determination of the LLA for a population is problematic. As noted previously, careful reconsideration of the early studies on autoregulation has resulted in a revised recommendation to maintain MAP at 70 mm Hg or higher in major anesthesia texts [6]. This number was derived from the mean LLA of the studies examined by Drummond in his brief review [38]. It has always been standard practice in articles to list the mean values with the standard deviations (SDs). As an unintended consequence of this practice, the focus of the data lies with the mean values, which when used as a cutoff point will not encompass a large proportion of the subjects and their variability. Using the mean value plus 1 SD should encompass 68.2% of the values in a normally distributed bell-shaped curve; the mean value plus 2 SDs, 95.9%; and the mean value plus 3 SDs, 99.7%. Drummond attempted to rectify this misconstrued extrapolation of autoregulation studies by denoting the ranges of the LLAs within multiple autoregulation studies in awake patients, instead of using only the mean LLAs (Box 3) [38]. The range of mean LLAs was 57 to 91 mm Hg, with 5 of these 7 studies obtaining a mean LLA of 70 mm Hg or higher. Moreover, if the ranges of LLAs within studies were examined, every study had the upper range of LLA above 70 mm Hg, and 4 of the 7 studies had the upper range of LLA at 100 mm Hg or higher. Notably, these autoregulation studies were performed in awake individuals, and presumably $CMRO_2$ will be reduced in patients under general anesthesia. Further, many of our anesthetic agents are cerebral vasodilators and may provide another "buffer" to preventing inadequate cerebral perfusion; yet, unfavorable physiologic conditions, which lower CBF or raise the LLA, such as hypocapnia and anemia, may also be present, which may decrease the margin for "error" or harm on lowering the blood pressure.

Defining LLA as a percentage reduction of MAP below baseline

Drummond [38] advocated revisiting what we considered a "safe" LLA by using percentage reductions from baseline resting MAPs as a way to address the extreme interpatient variability in absolute LLA values. This practice is standard management in neuroanesthesia. Strandgaard [39] demonstrated in 1976 that awake normotensive subjects' mean LLA was approximately 74% ± 12% of baseline, or a 26% ± 12% reduction from baseline MAP. In patients with uncontrolled hypertension, the LLA was 79% ± 10% of baseline MAP, or a 21% ± 10% reduction from baseline MAP (see Box 3). Ischemic symptoms developed in both groups at approximately 55% of baseline MAP, or a 45% reduction.

These percent reductions for LLAs are consistent with the recent nested case-control study of Bijker and colleagues [3], who studied more than 48,000 patients retrospectively and identified 42 patients with an ischemic stroke within 10 days of surgery. These stroke cases were matched by age and type of surgery to 252 control patients and adjusted for potential confounding factors. They found a statistically significant association with the duration that the intraoperative MAP was

Box 3: The lower limit of autoregulation

After reexamination of multiple autoregulation studies, the LLA has been shifted upward to 70 mm Hg in major texts.

This LLA will not encompass all patients, as there is tremendous interindividual variability in the LLA. Using a percent reduction from the baseline blood pressure as a method to estimate the LLA may accommodate this variability.

decreased more than 30% from baseline and the occurrence of an ischemic stroke within 10 days after surgery [3]; however, half of these 42 patients with stroke had carotid endarterectomy surgery and 6 had surgery for tumors of the head and neck. Only 13 cases of stroke occurred after general surgical procedures.

In sharp contrast to the previously mentioned work on the LLA are the multiple studies from Sharrock and colleagues [40] demonstrating that MAPs of 50 to 55 mm Hg are well tolerated by patients undergoing hip surgery in the lateral decubitus position using epidural local anesthetic infusions and intravenous epinephrine infusions. Early studies by this group without the epinephrine infusions had a "number of patients" with symptoms of cerebral ischemia, such as yawning, nausea, or drowsiness associated with cardiac indices lower than 1.8 L/min/m^2. When the low-dose epinephrine infusions were added, cardiac output was increased with a similar MAP, and the symptoms of cerebral ischemia abated. These studies imply that cardiac output either directly or indirectly affects CBF, as CPP reportedly stayed constant.

EFFECT OF SIMULTANEOUS FACTORS ON CBF: CLINICAL SCENARIOS

Patient condition and anesthetic management impose multiple simultaneous factors that can affect CBF, $CMRO_2$, cerebrovascular reactivity, and autoregulation. Consideration of the underlying vascular tone and the severity of the physiologic condition and dosage of anesthetic should be made when assessing adequacy of cerebral perfusion (Box 4). This section provides several examples of the effects of multiple simultaneous factors on CBF.

Effect of carbon dioxide on autoregulation in awake and anesthetized subjects

Baseline autoregulation studies are typically performed at $Paco_2$ of approximately 40 mm Hg, and they demonstrate the range of blood pressure over which an individual can alter their cerebrovascular tone to maintain a constant CBF. Because CO_2 also alters the vascular tone, at higher $Paco_2$ levels it will impose underlying vasodilation and alter the ability of the vasculature to further dilate with low MAP. Aaslid and colleagues [41] used transcranial Doppler and insonation of the middle cerebral artery in awake humans to demonstrate that the fastest rate of regulation of CBF velocity using thigh cuff deflation occurred with hypocapnia ($Paco_2$ of 22.2 mm Hg, highest tone) and the slowest with hypercapnia ($Paco_2$ of 46.9 mm Hg, lowest tone) [41]. At even higher $Paco_2$ levels (50–61 mm Hg) under remifentanil plus sevoflurane anesthesia (1.0%–1.1% end tidal concentration), McCulloch and colleagues [42], using transcranial Doppler, demonstrated that autoregulation

Box 4: Underlying vascular tone affects response on CBF

The effect of any drug or change in physiology on the CBF will depend on the underlying cerebrovascular tone.

was significantly impaired in healthy subjects. For propofol (140 μg/kg/min) anesthesia, the level at which significant impairment of autoregulation occurred was slightly higher, Pa_{CO_2} of 54 to 66 mm Hg. These findings are consistent with the concept of underlying vascular tone, in this case vasodilation, affecting the ability of the cerebral vessels to vasoconstrict. Moreover, McCulloch and colleagues [42] found that CO_2 reactivity was greater at an MAP of 100 mm Hg than at 80 mm Hg, for both sevoflurane and propofol, presumably because the underlying vasoconstriction at higher MAP allowed the CO_2 to exert a greater effect on vasodilation. At lower MAP with hypercapnia, the ability to vasodilate fully will be diminished compared with isocapnic conditions, and the LLA will be shifted to the right, or increased.

Effect of hypotension on carbon dioxide reactivity

Harper and Glass [43] demonstrated the effect of varying levels of hypotension on CO_2 reactivity in dogs anesthetized with nitrous oxide and oxygen and intermittent small doses of thiopentone (Fig. 4). With severe hypotension

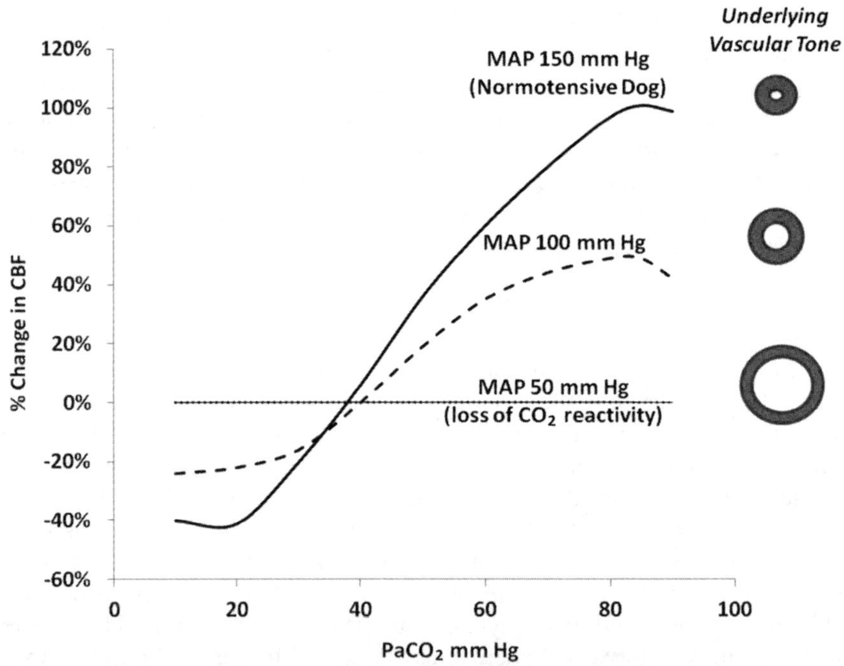

Fig. 4. The effect of hypotension on CO_2 reactivity in dogs. In normothermic (T 38°C), normotensive (MAP 150 mm Hg) dogs, the effect of CO_2 on CBF was almost linear between Pa_{CO_2} 20 to 80 mm Hg. The slope of the CO_2 reactivity curve decreases with moderate hypotension (MAP 100 mm Hg). CO_2 reactivity is abolished with severe hypotension at a MAP of 50 mm Hg because of the maximal underlying cerebrovascular dilation caused by the hypotension. (*Adapted from* Harper AM, Glass HI. Effect of alterations in the arterial carbon dioxide tension on the blood flow through the cerebral cortex at normal and low arterial blood pressures. J Neurol Neurosurg Psychiatry 1965;28:449.)

(via exsanguination) at a MAP of 50 mm Hg (normotensive MAP 150 mm Hg), CO_2 reactivity is abolished in the dog. The cerebral vasculature is presumably maximally vasodilated and cannot respond further to increasing $Paco_2$. The clinical implication is that during severe hypotension, raising the $Paco_2$ level will not necessarily increase CBF.

Effect of temperature and propofol dose on CBF and $CMRO_2$

Hypothermia (35°C) and increasing propofol doses in monkeys have additive effects on $CMRO_2$ and CBF reduction (Fig. 5) [44]. No significant interaction was found between temperature and propofol dose. These findings are consistent with other data suggesting that initial reductions in temperature exert a greater effect on basal metabolism, whereas anesthetic drugs exert their effect on functional metabolism. These additive reductions in $CMRO_2$ and CBF, with good flow-metabolism coupling, may be clinically useful in situations with elevated ICP.

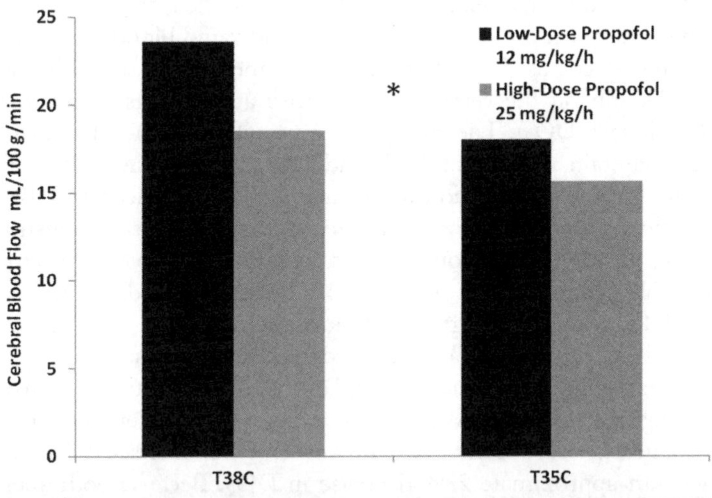

Fig. 5. The additive effects of mild hypothermia and propofol on CBF in dogs. Both propofol and mild hypothermia (35°C) decrease CBF and $CMRO_2$ with good flow-metabolism coupling in normothermic, isocapnic dogs. The effects are additive (no interaction effect), as mild hypothermia is thought to predominately affect basal metabolism and propofol affects functional metabolism. *$P<.05$ comparing normothermic with hypothermic propofol groups. (*Adapted from* Ouchi T, Ochiai R, Takeda J, et al. Combined effects of propofol and mild hypothermia on cerebral metabolism and blood flow in rhesus monkey: a positron emission tomography study. J Anesth 2006:20:208.)

Effect of anemia on CBF and autoregulation

Anemia increases CBF by 2 mechanisms, as discussed previously: reduced CaO_2 and reduced viscosity. Because the cerebral vessels are dilated with anemia, the LLA is shifted to the right. The ability of the cerebral vessels to dilate is limited because of the preexisting dilation caused by the anemia. Maruyama and colleagues [45] demonstrated that increasing severity of anemia (hematocrit values of 40%, 20%, and 5%) in dogs progressively raises the CBF at a MAP of 100 mm Hg, such that CBF with a hematocrit of 20% is 1.7-fold that of baseline hematocrit of 40%, and CBF with a hematocrit of 5% is 3.0-fold higher than baseline. Additionally, the range of autoregulatory capacity is progressively diminished with increasing severity of anemia and the LLA is shifted to the right. The first point of significant CBF reduction in the studies by Maruyama and colleagues [45], tested at 20–mm Hg increments from MAP 100 to MAP 40 mm Hg, was 40 mm Hg with hematocrit 40%, 60 mm Hg with hematocrit 20%, and 80 mm Hg with hematocrit 5%. These findings may have significant clinical implications for patients in the intensive care unit with stenotic neurovascular lesions or acute neurologic injuries with or without elevated ICP, where current practice is to avoid transfusion and to tolerate very low hematocrits.

Effect of anemia and hypotension on CBF and O_2 delivery

During major surgical procedures with large and rapid blood loss, anemia and hypotension may coexist. As noted previously, anemia will superimpose underlying vasodilation on the cerebral vasculature and increase CBF to provide stable O_2 delivery (DO_2). The ability of the vessels to further dilate with hypotension to maintain a constant CBF and DO_2 will be diminished. Previous experiments from our institution using microspheres to measure CBF in normocapnic, normothermic pigs anesthetized with isoflurane demonstrated this concept (Fig. 6) [46]. One group of pigs was made hypotensive (euvolemic) with labetalol (MAP from 73 mm Hg to 52 mm Hg) and maintained stable CBF and DO_2. A separate group of normotensive pigs was made anemic (hematocrit from 27% to 17% with shed blood and crystalloid replacement to maintain euvolemia) and increased CBF by approximately 50% from baseline, resulting in stable DO_2. When the conditions of both euvolemic hypotension and anemia were combined, however, CBF increased by only 8%, resulting in an approximate 28% decrease in DO_2. Because both anemia and hypotension require cerebral vasodilation to maintain a stable DO_2, the combined effects overwhelmed the capacity of the cerebral vasculature to vasodilate sufficiently, thereby decreasing DO_2. Clinical implications are that patients with severe anemia may not be able to compensate for very low blood pressure to maintain stable DO_2 to the brain. These findings have implications for limiting the extremes of anemia and hypotension when attempting to minimize blood loss and/or avoid transfusion.

ANESTHETIC DRUGS AND VASOACTIVE AGENTS

This section discusses pharmacologic agents available to clinicians to help optimize cerebral perfusion, $CMRO_2$, and brain relaxation in everyday practice. Because many of the vasoactive drugs are used to lower blood pressure, results may affected when MAP falls outside of the LLA.

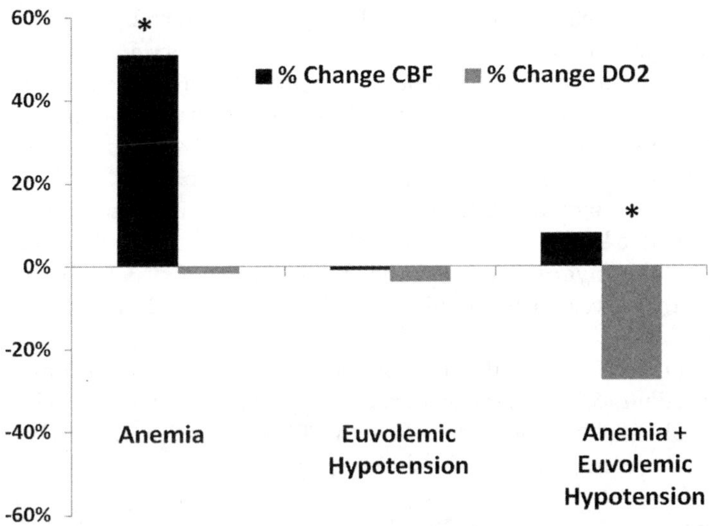

Fig. 6. The effects of anemia and hypotension on CBF and O_2 delivery. In normocapnic, normothermic pigs anesthetized with isoflurane, anemia resulted in a dramatic increase in CBF, which kept the O_2 delivery (DO_2) to the brain stable. Similarly, severe hypotension to a MAP of approximately 50 mm Hg, resulted in stable CBF and stable DO_2. When both conditions were combined, the CBF increased only 8%, resulting in a 28% drop in DO_2 (*$P<.05$). The degree of vasodilation by the cerebral vasculature is limited and may not provide stable DO_2 under extreme physiologic conditions. (*Adapted from* Lee LA, Deem S, Glenny RW, et al. Effects of anemia and hypotension on porcine optic nerve blood flow and oxygen delivery. Anesthesiology 2008;108(5):864.)

Calcium channel blockers

In general, calcium channel blockers (CCBs) exert their effect by inhibiting the influx of intracellular calcium via voltage-gated calcium channels on the membrane of the sarcoplasmic reticulum. This inhibition results in less intracellular calcium available, leading to a weaker contraction. CCBs can be divided into 2 categories based on the presence or absence of a dihydropyridine group. Dihydropyridine drugs include amlodipine, clevidipine, felodipine, nicardipine, nifedipine, and nimodipine, whereas nondihydropyridine drugs include diltiazem and verapamil. Calcium channels are morphologically distinct in different types of tissue, including the brain, myocardium, vascular smooth muscle, and the atrioventricular (AV) conduction system. Thus, there is intraclass variability with regard to binding selectivity of each calcium channel blocker [47].

Although most of the dihydropyridines exhibit activity in all vascular smooth muscle, decreasing cardiac afterload and providing a generalized hypotensive effect, nimodipine shows relative selectivity to the cerebral arteries at clinical doses [48]. It has been shown to provide clinical effectiveness in treating vasospasm following subarachnoid hemorrhage in humans [49]. Accordingly, a hypotensive effect is less common with nimodipine, and there is evidence that nimodipine slightly increases CBF and cerebral metabolic rate [50]. The other dihydropyridines tend to act mainly in the periphery and have no specific effect on CBF and cerebral metabolic rate provided mean arterial pressure is kept constant [51]. Nicardipine is one of the most commonly used intravenous CCBs in the neurosurgical patient because of its ease of titration. Clevidipine, approved by the Food and Drug Administration in 2008, is degraded by plasma esterases with a half-life of approximately 1 minute, compared with nicardipine with a half-life of 4 to 5 hours [52]. Nondihydropyridine CCBs generally act on the myocardium and the AV conduction system, but also have a small cerebral vasodilatory effect with increases in CBF, and thus potential to increase ICP.

CCBs may also block the accumulation of intracellular calcium, which is involved in intracellular signaling processes in neuronal injury. Unfortunately, clinical trials have not shown benefit with CCBs, and some experts believe that more downstream pathways should be targeted [53].

NO donors

NO donors represent another class of drugs that can be therapeutically useful to treat acute episodes of hypertension, but these drugs have their own side effects that must be considered. All NO donors release NO in the vasculature, which then activates intracellular guanylate cyclase and increases intracellular production of cyclic guanosine monophosphate (GMP). Cyclic GMP, in turn, activates protein kinase G that inactivates myosin light chains causing smooth muscle relaxation and resultant vasodilation. The cerebral vasodilation caused by the NO donor drugs can result in significant increases in ICP.

Nitroprusside comes as a salt (sodium nitroprusside [SNP]) and for each molecule of NO that is released, there remains a potential 5 cyanide ions that can also be released and cause toxicity within 2 to 3 hours [54]. Studies on cerebral hemodynamics with SNP show variable results depending on study conditions but, for the most part, it has little effect on CBF in anesthetized neurosurgical patients [55]. Larger doses have been associated with loss of autoregulation, decreased CBF, and increased ICP. Recognizing the aforementioned concerns, the exceptionally short half-life of 3 to 4 minutes makes SNP useful when used on a short-term basis for acute control of blood pressure.

Nitroglycerin preferentially works as a venodilator and only affects arterial tone at higher clinical doses in a somewhat unpredictable way. Nitroglycerin has been shown to vasodilate the major cerebral vessels and to cause a decrease in CBF velocity but no change in CBF [56]. Other studies have shown a profound increase in ICP and decrease in CPP with nitroglycerin [57]. Hydralazine, also an NO donor, has its effects mainly at the level of the arterioles with vasodilation. It has similar effects in the brain and the periphery, causing cerebral vasodilation, increased CBF, and increased ICP.

Adenosine has direct vasodilating effects in the brain, and intravenous infusion will cause vasodilation of the major cerebral vessels, but no change in CBF [58].

It causes transient heart block (and subsequent cardiac arrest in higher doses) and is used intraoperatively to transiently stop CBF to facilitate clipping of cerebral aneurysms.

Sympatholytics and sympathomimetics

Whether or not drugs that stimulate or antagonize the body's intrinsic sympathetic nerve system affect CBF and autoregulation depends on the starting blood pressure, the clinical dose of the drug given, whether autoregulation is already impaired, and if the blood brain barrier is open or closed [6]. As a rule, sympatholytics and sympathomimetics do not have any major direct effects on CBF outside of their effects on systemic blood pressure, with a few exceptions that will be discussed in the following paragraphs.

Alpha-1 agonists are frequently used in patients with shock and are commonly administered to patients undergoing anesthesia. Although there is potential concern with alpha agonists causing further vasoconstriction leading to decreased CBF, there is not sufficient evidence to suggest this is the case in humans. Intracarotid infusion of norepinephrine has been shown to have no effect on CBF [6], and phenylephrine has been shown not to decrease CBF intraoperatively while patients are on cardiopulmonary bypass [59]. At clinical doses, norepinephrine does carry some beta activity, which gives it different characteristics with respect to cerebral perfusion than phenylephrine.

Alpha-2 agonists used in clinical practice are clonidine and dexmedetomidine, the latter of which shows much higher specificity to the alpha-2 adrenoreceptor. Dexmedetomidine has been shown to decrease $CMRO_2$ and CBF [60,61].

Beta agonists in lower concentrations have few direct effects on the cerebral vasculature, but in higher doses can increase $CMRO_2$ and CBF [62]. This effect seems to be pronounced when there is a compromise in the blood brain barrier, suggesting a direct effect of beta agonists on cerebral metabolic rate [63].

It has become clear that beta-blockers in clinical use today can be thought of in 2 categories: beta antagonists and beta inverse agonists [64]. Beta agonists cause an increase in $CMRO_2$, and thus CBF. Beta-blockers demonstrate either no effect or a reduction in CBF [6]. Esmolol, a fast-acting beta blocker with a short half-life, has been shown to decrease anesthetic requirements, suggesting it may also decrease $CMRO_2$ and demonstrate some inverse agonist activity in the brain [65,66].

Dopamine has also been studied extensively and used mainly as a vasopressor in certain disease states, mainly to increase blood pressure in the intensive care setting in septic shock and certain types of cerebral ischemia. The medical literature currently suggests dopamine works well to increase CBF in other populations, such as preterm infants who are hypotensive [67] and patients with TBI [68], although it is not the agent of choice. In general, it has not demonstrated any direct effects on CBF, but does cause an increase in the $CMRO_2$ of the choroid plexus and basal ganglia [69,70].

Vasopressin, although not classically considered a part of the sympathetic nervous system, has mainly been studied in situations of cardiac arrest and very little has been contributed on lower-dose vasopressin therapy and its effect on CBF.

Intravenous anesthetic agents

Most intravenous anesthetic agents, with the exception of ketamine, cause a reduction in $CMRO_2$ and CBF, exhibiting flow-metabolism coupling. Propofol, barbiturates, and etomidate all directly cause a reduction in $CMRO_2$ by agonizing γ-aminobutyric acid (GABA) sites, with a resultant decrease in CBF and ICP. Ketamine, an N-methyl-D-aspartate receptor antagonist, increases $CMRO_2$, CBF, and ICP in awake subjects [71]. When ventilation is controlled to prevent a rise in $Paco_2$, and a background anesthetic is also given, such as a potent volatile anesthetic or a benzodiazepine, there is no increase in $CMRO_2$, CBF, or ICP.

Benzodiazepines appear also to produce a modest reduction in CBF, but to a lesser extent than seen with other GABA agonists. This is believed to be because of a reduction in CMR and a preservation of the coupling of CMR and CBF [5]. Opioids have shown variable responses in clinical studies and seem to depend on other anesthetics concomitantly given. In general, the effects, if present, tend to be mild and may not be clinically significant.

Volatile anesthetic agents

Volatile anesthetic agents differ from intravenous anesthetic agents in that they reduce $CMRO_2$ in a dose-dependent fashion, but increase CBF, particularly at concentrations greater than 1 minimum alveolar concentration. Halothane has a far greater effect on CBF than isoflurane, desflurane, or sevoflurane, which all have similar effects on cerebral vasodilation. NO and xenon vary from the halogenated anesthetics in their effects on CBF. NO is shown to increase CBF with a variable effect on $CMRO_2$ [72]. When used as an adjunct to intravenous anesthetics, NO causes little change in CBF; however, when it is used in conjunction with volatile anesthetics, it causes a more dramatic increase in CBF and ICP [72]. Xenon seems to show a differential effect on CBF on gray matter and white matter, causing a decrease in the former and increase in the latter [73].

In general, when considering the pharmacologic effect of a drug on cerebral perfusion, one must consider the drug's effects on the cerebral vasculature if this varies from its effect on the systemic vasculature, the drug's effect on cerebral metabolic rate, the blood pressure before giving the drug, whether or not administration of the drug will bring the blood pressure outside or inside the cerebral autoregulatory window, and the patient's condition with respect to CBF, $CMRO_2$, and ICP (Box 5).

PATIENT DISEASE STATES

Although understanding the complex nature of CBF and autoregulation is important, it is essential for a clinician to understand how to apply these concepts to an individual patient, especially when these complex mechanisms

Box 5: Pharmacology key points

- Pharmacologic mechanisms of optimizing cerebral perfusion include altering systemic arterial pressure, cerebral metabolic rate, and directly acting on cerebral arteries and arterioles.
- Drugs that can alter cerebral metabolic rate include not only anesthetics, but sympatholytics and sympathomimetics, especially when the blood brain barrier has been compromised.
- When considering an individual drug's effect on an individual patient, one must consider the patient's current condition and what other factors are already affecting CBF, cerebral metabolic rate, and ICP.
- There is some inconsistency in the medical literature with regard to individual drug effects on CBF, probably because of lack of control of type of anesthetic, anemia, etc. several other factors that also influence CBF such as (systemic MAP, CO_2 level, awake versus anesthetized, temperature, type of anesthetic.

are affected by patient disease, whether it be congenital abnormalities, acquired chronic disease, or acute injury (Box 6).

Anatomic variants

The most common relevant patient condition is one that will rarely be identified preoperatively, but can affect a patient's reserve for tolerating hemodynamic challenges. The anatomy of the circle of Willis varies widely in human populations, with estimates showing an intact circle of Willis in as low as 34% of the population [74–76]. There is evidence suggesting that patients with an anatomic variant of the classic circle of Willis will have different perfusion patterns and that some may be at higher risk for ischemia than others, particularly in the presence of acquired stenotic lesions [77–79].

There is significant evidence in the literature that patients with an incomplete circle of Willis, to the extent that limits collateral flow, carry a higher lifetime risk of stroke, particularly in the presence of carotid stenosis. This was best shown with prospective data from the North American Symptomatic Carotid Endarterectomy Trial (NASCET) [80], but also with retrospective data showing a nonfunctional anterior collateral pathway increased the risk of

Box 6: Patient disease state key points

- Subclinical anatomic abnormalities can make patients more susceptible to ischemic neurologic deficits perioperatively, particularly in the presence of stenotic vascular lesions.
- Certain disease states, such as hypertension, can shift the normal cerebral autoregulation curve to the right.
- TBI can impair normal autoregulation mechanisms making blood pressure control in these patients paramount to preventing secondary brain injury.

ischemic stroke by sevenfold [81]. Additionally, the absence of posterior communicating arteries, the channel that connects the anterior circulation with the posterior circulation, was associated with border zone infarcts [82], and the fetal-type circulation has also been associated with higher rates of stroke in the medical literature with retrospective data [83]. What remains challenging about treating patients with congenital defects is they are mostly subclinical until a neurologic insult has occurred.

Age effects

There are several common diseases that frequently accompany aging, such as cerebrovascular disease, cardiovascular disease, and neurologic disease, that each modify cerebral perfusion and autoregulation in their own way, but increasing age itself seems to have very little to no effect on dynamic autoregulation [84]. Older patients do have decreased baroreceptor sensitivity and a change in position could change CBF values significantly, but the autoregulation curve itself seems to be unaffected [85]. There is evidence that static autoregulation appears to be affected with increasing age [86]. Elderly patients also exhibit a wider range of blood pressures diurnally, and elderly patients may be subject to regional hypoperfusion during certain times of night [87]. Additionally, overall CBF decreases from childhood to middle age, which may reflect progressive neuronal loss over time [88].

At the other spectrum of age, premature infants are also a vulnerable population, as development and maturation of the cerebral vasculature usually is not complete. In premature infants weighing less than 1500 g, passive CBF is common, suggesting the autoregulatory mechanisms are still developing and are not working 20% of the time [89].

Chronic hypertension

Patients with chronic hypertension show structural changes in the cerebral circulation, such as vascular hypertrophy and a shift in the autoregulation curve to the right producing a higher threshold for the ULA [90]. Studies in rats provide evidence that these structural changes also provide somewhat of a protective effect on the HLA and allow chronically hypertensive patients to tolerate higher blood pressures without causing a hemorrhagic stroke. Because of these changes, acute hypotension induced with an NO donor, one of the human body's intrinsic mechanisms of vasodilation, is not tolerated as well in these patients and leads to decreased perfusion during hypotension when compared with normotensive subjects [91]. There is also evidence suggesting there are subclinical regional perfusion abnormalities in the untreated hypertensive patient [92].

Treating patients with chronic hypertension does provide benefit, as evidenced by a decreased rate of ischemic stroke [93,94] and a restoration of more normal CBF dynamics [95,96]. Acute and chronic care of the chronically hypertensive patient should be undertaken carefully using the pharmacologic principles mentioned previously that favor mechanisms causing cerebral vasodilation in addition to peripheral vasodilation.

Although most studies looking at the relationship of CBF and hypertension have been in adults, a growing prevalence of hypertension in the pediatric population urges the scientific community to examine this population more closely. It has already been shown that there is an association between hypertension and altered cerebral hemodynamics in children, potentially causing new problems in childhood not previously seen [97].

Carotid stenosis/occlusion

Carotid artery stenosis is a disease of plaque buildup associated with aging and hyperlipidemia. One main problem with the disease is that it typically remains subclinical until it has already progressed into advanced stages. Less commonly, carotid artery stenosis can develop as a complication of radiation therapy to the neck [98].

Carotid artery stenosis can lead to regional hypoperfusion if a patient's anatomy does not permit adequate collateral flow. According to analysis of the NASCET data, presence of collateral flow decreases subsequent stroke rate by as much as 60% [99]. Despite collateral flow, there is still a decrease in cerebrovascular reserve that correlates exponentially with increasing degrees of carotid stenosis [100]. The vasculature supplied by the affected carotid artery may lose its cerebrovascular reactivity [101]. Recently, investigators have found that occlusion of the external carotid artery on the same side may also increase stroke risk [102].

Although there has been much debate about when to surgically intervene with either a carotid endarterectomy or stenting, it is clear that these procedures can provide overall benefits in selected populations. Key deciding factors mainly include degree of stenosis and presence of neurologic symptoms. Procedures to alleviate carotid stenosis restore CBF and autoregulatory capacity to previously hypoperfused vasculature, and may improve some cognitive deficits induced by carotid artery stenosis [103,104].

There has been immense interest in determining the best course of treatment for carotid artery stenosis, whether it be placement of a carotid artery stent (CAS) or carotid endarterectomy (CEA). A randomized controlled trial of CAS versus CEA ("CREST" trial) demonstrated no statistically significant difference in the primary outcome (determined as combined rates of periprocedural mortality, myocardial infarction, and stroke, and ipsilateral stroke over 4 years) between the 2 groups; however, the rate of stroke (4.1% vs 2.3%, $P = .012$) was higher with CAS, whereas the rate of myocardial infarction was slightly higher with CEA (1.1% vs 2.3%, $P = .032$) [105]. Additionally, outcomes for patients younger than 70 years were better with CAS, and outcomes were better with CEA for patients older than 70 years or with symptomatic stenosis. Since publication of the CREST trial and some meta-analyses following it, the American Heart Association and American Stroke Association published collaborative recommendations indicating carotid endarterectomy for symptomatic patients and for older patients, and carotid artery stenting for certain asymptomatic patients of younger age [106].

Cerebral hyperperfusion syndrome (CHS) can occur after a symptom-free interval postoperatively in 1% to 3% of patients, and is thought to be caused by an impaired autoregulatory mechanism in the affected hypoperfused tissue that takes time to recover after normal flow is restored [107–109]. It can occur up to 4 weeks after the original procedure and is associated with a symptomatic period of nausea, vomiting, headache, or other neurologic deficits. If untreated, it may lead to ipsilateral hemorrhagic stroke and death in up to 40% of patients [107]. Methods recently proposed to help prevent this complication, in addition to strict perioperative blood pressure control, include staged angioplasty, perioperative transcranial Doppler measurements, and calculating cerebral circulation time.

Traumatic brain injury

TBI is a substantial public health problem with approximately 1.7 million TBIs every year in the United States [110]. Although the most effective treatment for this disease is prevention, most medical intervention is focused around preventing secondary injury, which can affect all systems of the body. Understanding how cerebral perfusion and autoregulation can be altered in these patients is paramount to preventing secondary brain injury.

In addition to preventing common sequelae of TBI that negatively affect the brain, such as hypotension, hypoxia, hypoglycemia, hyperthermia, hypocapnia, and intracranial hypertension, the main focus of treatment of TBI is to continuously deliver oxygen to the brain, which is done by optimizing CPP, as autoregulation is frequently impaired even with mild head injuries. There have been several new methods recently published determining methods of tailoring therapy to each individual patient's "ideal perfusion pressure" by analyzing ICP waveforms in addition to arterial pressure waveforms, respiratory oscillations, transcranial Doppler, and, in some cases, short-term moderate hypocapnia [111–113]. In addition, optimizing and measuring neuronal tissue oxygenation may improve neurologic outcome [114].

In pediatric patients in whom normal CPP values vary widely depending on age, recent research has focused on the pressure reactivity index to determine the ideal CPP in children. It is being used to correlate mortality with pressures below the ideal pressure, and disability with pressures above the ideal pressure [115]. It may prove to be an important therapeutic target, as low CBF and poor autoregulatory capacity are highly correlated with poor outcomes [116].

EFFECTS OF POSITIONING ON CEREBRAL PERFUSION

Surgery in the beach chair position

A controversial topic surrounding cerebral perfusion that has arisen in the past several years is anesthetic management of blood pressure in the beach chair position in patients receiving general anesthesia. This concern arose after a series of 4 cases was reported in 2005, detailing severe brain damage in the beach chair position for shoulder surgery [117]. These devastating injuries were thought to be the result of both surgical requests for deliberate hypotension and lack of correction of the blood pressure in the sitting position for height from the noninvasive blood pressure (NIBP) cuff to the external auditory meatus (EAC). Although measuring blood pressure at the EAC has always been standard practice in neuroanesthesia, this concept did not effectively transmit into other surgical arenas, particularly one known for relatively minor outpatient procedures.

Correcting the blood pressure to account for height difference between the site of measurement and the brain addresses the hydrostatic gradient from the effect of gravity (Fig. 7). For every centimeter of height difference between the NIBP cuff and the EAC, 0.77 mm Hg should be subtracted from the NIBP reading on the arm or leg to approximate the true MAP at the EAC (or for every inch difference, 2 mm Hg subtracted). It is based on the theory that the cerebral circulation acts similar to a "waterfall" system subject to gravitational effects, rather than as a closed siphon system that operates independent of gravity. Since this case series and subsequent controversy, an experiment in anesthetized giraffes demonstrated that the CBF was controlled by arterial pressure without contribution from a siphon mechanism [118]. Admittedly, the waterfall concept does not fully explain cerebral circulation in instances of zero gravity; yet it appears to account for clinically relevant situations.

Many clinical studies have also been performed since this case series was published, including McCulloch and colleagues' [119] study showing that MAP at the EAC decreased 47% ± 7% in the sitting position at 45° with an associated 22% ± 7% decrease in the CBF velocity in the middle cerebral artery. Systolic blood pressure was 96 ± 10 mm Hg by noninvasive measurement on the arm. Another study, by Jeong and colleagues [120], demonstrated jugular desaturation to less than 50% for at least 5 minutes in 41% of patients in the beach chair position under general anesthesia, with a significantly higher proportion of desaturations in the propofol/remifentanil group (56%) compared with the sevoflurane/50% NO group (21%, $P = .008$). Jugular saturation in the sitting position in the propofol/remifentanil group decreased by 22% ± 12% from supine baseline, and by 14% ± 12% in the sevoflurane/50% NO group.

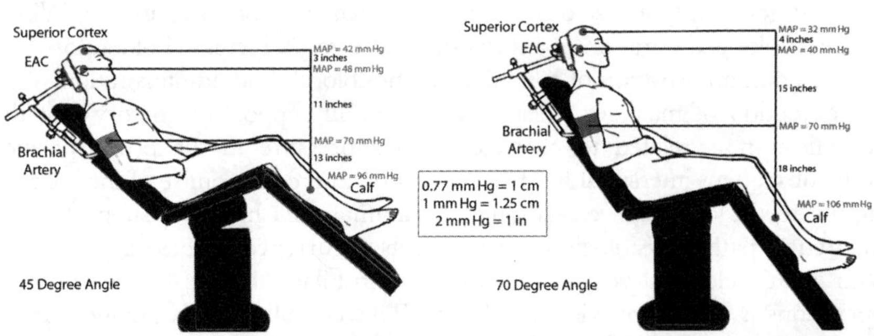

Fig. 7. Beach chair position shown at 45° angle on left, and 70° angle on right. MAP calculations shown when correcting for the hydrostatic gradient from the site of the noninvasive blood pressure measurement to the brain.

Jugular desaturation was also related to MAP lower than 50 mm Hg measured at the EAC.

One practice that may further place these patients at risk for cerebral ischemia is the frequent surgical request for deliberate hypotension, particularly when it is facilitated with drugs that do not cause cerebral vasodilation. In addition to the need to correct for the hydrostatic gradient in these cases, we previously discussed how hypotension caused by low cardiac output (ie, hemorrhage, or in this situation head up position under general anesthesia) has been shown to raise the LLA compared with hypotension induced by vasoactive agents. Other issues that may predispose to inadequate cerebral perfusion are the wide variability in the LLA among individuals, the very high incidence of incomplete circle of Willis anatomy in the general population, specialized headrests and head positions that may distort the vascular anatomy in the head and neck, and previously asymptomatic stenotic vascular lesions. Despite having the "deck" stacked against adequate cerebral perfusion in these procedures, the incidence of these devastating injuries appears to be low, although no reliable mechanism for reporting exists. These procedures are typically brief, lasting only a few hours; yet, one professional liability company recently noted at least 9 lawsuits associated with neurological injuries sustained in the beach chair position with large settlement payments related to the issue of hypotension and uncorrected blood pressure in the sitting position [121].

Venous effect on CPP: ischemic optic neuropathy associated with prolonged prone or steep trendelenburg position

Since the late 1990s, the perioperative complication of ischemic optic neuropathy after prolonged prone spine surgery has received significant attention from anesthesiologists, spine surgeons, and neuro-ophthalmologists. In early 2012, a multicenter case-control study using 80 cases of ischemic optic neuropathy (ION) from the American Society of Anesthesiologists Postoperative Visual Loss Registry and comparing them with 315 controls from 17 centers across North America identified 6 independent risk factors for ION after prone spine surgery [122]. These 6 risk factors are male sex, obesity, use of a Wilson frame, prolonged duration of anesthesia (ie, surgery), increased blood loss, and decreased administration of colloid in the nonblood fluid administration. With the exception of male sex, these risk factors all support the theory that this complication is related to elevated venous pressure in the prone position with subsequent interstitial fluid accumulation and compromise of the vascular supply to the optic nerve. Although no animal data have yet supported this theoretical pathophysiologic mechanism, its occurrence in these 2 procedures with greatly elevated venous pressure, and in bilateral radical head and neck operations is consistent with this theory. This complication is unique because it highlights the importance of outflow pressure in CPP in non-neurosurgical procedures. Whether or not increasing the MAP in these cases is beneficial has not been tested, as it is not clear that using excessive inflow pressure will improve perfusion once the venous outflow problem has developed. Interestingly, these patients often do not have associated cerebral injuries. Currently, there is no reliable intraoperative monitor for detecting optic nerve ischemia or dysfunction intraoperatively during general anesthesia.

INTRAOPERATIVE MONITORS FOR ASSESSMENT OF CBF AND CEREBRAL ISCHEMIA

For the general anesthesiologist, use of equipment such as a transcranial Doppler, although useful, is not practical, and can require significant setup time. For high-risk cases, such as CEA, its benefit may be enormous, and obtaining a vascular technologist to measure CBF velocity intraoperatively is recommended when available. Similarly, 16-channel EEG is not likely to be used on an outpatient procedure, but may prove valuable in high-risk procedures. Alternatively, the widespread use of the bispectral index, which is a processed EEG, can provide crude assessments of frontal brain activity, and may give some indication of global adequacy of perfusion. Near infrared spectroscopy is currently widely used in research, but its reliance on trends and lack of absolute values for ischemia make its validity unclear, particularly in adults in whom skull thickness is much greater than in neonates. For anesthesiologists who work at major neurosurgical or neurotrauma centers, familiarity with ICP monitors is essential, and use of surgically placed brain tissue oxygen monitors and autoregulation testing may also be useful for guiding anesthetic management. The expansion of intraoperative evoked potential monitoring to detect cerebral ischemia, as well as injury to the spinal cord and peripheral nerves, may significantly alter anesthetic management, and can provide early warnings of injury and allow modification of surgical and anesthetic care.

The concepts discussed in this updated review should help anesthesiologists optimize management of cerebral perfusion in routine outpatient and inpatient procedures, high-risk neurosurgical and non-neurosurgical procedures, and in high-risk patients with preexisting cerebrovascular disease.

References

[1] Mashour GA, Shanks AM, Kheterpal S. Perioperative stroke and associated mortality after noncardiac, nonneurologic surgery. Anesthesiology 2011;114(6):1289–96.

[2] Devereaux PJ, Yang H, Yusuf S, et al. Effects of extended-release metoprolol succinate in patients undergoing non-cardiac surgery (POISE trial): a randomised controlled trial. Lancet 2008;371(9627):1839–47.

[3] Bijker JB, Persoon S, Peelen LM, et al. Intraoperative hypotension and perioperative ischemic stroke after general surgery: a nested case-control study. Anesthesiology 2012;116(3):658–64.

[4] Ng JL, Chan MT, Gelb AW. Perioperative stroke in noncardiac, nonneurosurgical surgery. Anesthesiology 2011;115(4):879–90.

[5] Cottrell JE, Young WL. Cottrell's neuroanesthesia. 5th edition. St. Louis (MO); London: Mosby; 2009.

[6] Miller RD. Miller's anesthesia. 7th edition. Philadelphia: Churchhill Livingstone Elsevier; 2010.

[7] Bell BA. A history of the study of the cerebral circulation and the measurement of cerebral blood flow. Neurosurgery 1984;14(2):238–46.

[8] Jakovcevic D, Harder DR. Role of astrocytes in matching blood flow to neuronal activity. Curr Top Dev Biol 2007;79:75–97.
[9] Gordon GR, Howarth C, MacVicar BA. Bidirectional control of arteriole diameter by astrocytes. Exp Physiol 2011;96(4):393–9.
[10] Iliff JJ, Wang R, Zeldin DC, et al. Epoxyeicosanoids as mediators of neurogenic vasodilation in cerebral vessels. Am J Physiol Heart Circ Physiol 2009;296(5): H1352–63.
[11] Kety SS, Schmidt CF. The effects of altered arterial tensions of carbon dioxide and oxygen on cerebral blood flow and cerebral oxygen consumption of normal young men. J Clin Invest 1948;27(4):484–92.
[12] Iliff LD, Zilkha E, Du Boulay GH, et al. Cerebrovascular carbon dioxide reactivity and conductance in patients awake and under general anesthesia. Neurology 1976;26(9): 835–8.
[13] Lindauer U, Vogt J, Schuh-Hofer S, et al. Cerebrovascular vasodilation to extraluminal acidosis occurs via combined activation of ATP-sensitive and Ca2+-activated potassium channels. J Cereb Blood Flow Metab 2003;23(10):1227–38.
[14] Wagerle LC, Degiulio PA. Indomethacin-sensitive CO2 reactivity of cerebral arterioles is restored by vasodilator prostaglandin. Am J Phys 1994;266(4 Pt 2):H1332–8.
[15] Gupta AK, Menon DK, Czosnyka M, et al. Thresholds for hypoxic cerebral vasodilation in volunteers. Anesth Analg 1997;85(4):817–20.
[16] Borgstrom L, Johannsson H, Siesjo BK. The relationship between arterial po2 and cerebral blood flow in hypoxic hypoxia. Acta Physiol Scand 1975;93(3):423–32.
[17] Van Mil AH, Spilt A, Van Buchem MA, et al. Nitric oxide mediates hypoxia-induced cerebral vasodilation in humans. J Appl Phys 2002;92(3):962–6.
[18] Todd MM, Farrell S, Wu B. Cerebral blood flow during hypoxemia and hemodilution in rabbits: different roles for nitric oxide? J Cereb Blood Flow Metab 1997;17(12): 1319–25.
[19] Vavilala MS, Lee LA, Morris GP, et al. Cerebral autoregulation before and after blood transfusion in a child. J Neurosurg Anesthesiol 2001;13(3):233–6.
[20] Tomiyama Y, Jansen K, Brian JE Jr, et al. Hemodilution, cerebral O2 delivery, and cerebral blood flow: a study using hyperbaric oxygenation. Am J Phys 1999;276(4 Pt 2):H1190–6.
[21] Clifton GL, Miller ET, Choi SC, et al. Lack of effect of induction of hypothermia after acute brain injury. N Engl J Med 2001;344(8):556–63.
[22] Todd MM, Hindman BJ, Clarke WR, et al. Mild intraoperative hypothermia during surgery for intracranial aneurysm. N Engl J Med 2005;352(2):135–45.
[23] Arrich J, Holzer M, Havel C, et al. Hypothermia for neuroprotection in adults after cardiopulmonary resuscitation. Cochrane Database Syst Rev 2012;9:CD004128.
[24] Cremer OL, Diephuis JC, van Soest H, et al. Cerebral oxygen extraction and autoregulation during extracorporeal whole body hyperthermia in humans. Anesthesiology 2004;100(5):1101–7.
[25] Fan JL, Cotter JD, Lucas RA, et al. Human cardiorespiratory and cerebrovascular function during severe passive hyperthermia: effects of mild hypohydration. J Appl Phys 2008;105(2):433–45.
[26] Peterson EC, Wang Z, Britz G. Regulation of cerebral blood flow. Int J Vasc Med 2011;2011:823525.
[27] Cassaglia PA, Griffiths RI, Walker AM. Sympathetic nerve activity in the superior cervical ganglia increases in response to imposed increases in arterial pressure. Am J Physiol Regul Integr Comp Physiol 2008;294(4):R1255–61.
[28] Hernandez MJ, Raichle ME, Stone HL. The role of the sympathetic nervous system in cerebral blood flow autoregulation. Eur Neurol 1971;6(1):175–9.
[29] Heistad DD. Summary of symposium on cerebral blood flow: effect of nerves and neurotransmitters. Cardiovascular center, University of Iowa, Iowa City, Iowa, June 16–18, 1981. J Cereb Blood Flow Metab 1981;1(4):447–50.

[30] D'Alecy LG. Relation between sympathetic cerebral vasoconstriction and CSF pressure. Eur Neurol 1971;6(1):180–4.
[31] Fitch W, Ferguson GG, Sengupta D, et al. Autoregulation of cerebral blood flow during controlled hypotension in baboons. J Neurol Neurosurg Psychiatr 1976;39(10):1014–22.
[32] Jones SC, Easley KA, Radinsky CR, et al. Nitric oxide synthase inhibition depresses the height of the cerebral blood flow-pressure autoregulation curve during moderate hypotension. J Cereb Blood Flow Metab 2003;23(9):1085–95.
[33] Finnerty FA Jr, Witkin L, Fazekas JF. Cerebral hemodynamics during cerebral ischemia induced by acute hypotension. J Clin Invest 1954;33(9):1227–32.
[34] Sharbrough FW, Messick JM Jr, Sundt TM Jr. Correlation of continuous electroencephalograms with cerebral blood flow measurements during carotid endarterectomy. Stroke 1973;4(4):674–83.
[35] Branston NM, Ladds A, Symon L, et al. Comparison of the effects of ischaemia on early components of the somatosensory evoked potential in brainstem, thalamus, and cerebral cortex. J Cereb Blood Flow Metab 1984;4(1):68–81.
[36] Leech PJ, Miller JD, Fitch W, et al. Cerebral blood flow, internal carotid artery pressure, and the EEG as a guide to the safety of carotid ligation. J Neurol Neurosurg Psychiatr 1974;37(7):854–62.
[37] Astrup J, Symon L, Branston NM, et al. Cortical evoked potential and extracellular K+ and H+ at critical levels of brain ischemia. Stroke 1977;8(1):51–7.
[38] Drummond JC. The lower limit of autoregulation: time to revise our thinking? Anesthesiology 1997;86(6):1431–3.
[39] Strandgaard S. Autoregulation of cerebral blood flow in hypertensive patients. The modifying influence of prolonged antihypertensive treatment on the tolerance to acute, drug-induced hypotension. Circulation 1976;53(4):720–7.
[40] Sharrock NE, Mineo R, Urquhart B. Hemodynamic response to low-dose epinephrine infusion during hypotensive epidural anesthesia for total hip replacement. Reg Anesth 1990;15(6):295–9.
[41] Aaslid R, Lindegaard KF, Sorteberg W, et al. Cerebral Autoregulation Dynamics in Humans. Stroke 1989;20(1):45–52.
[42] McCulloch TJ, Visco E, Lam AM. Graded hypercapnia and cerebral autoregulation during sevoflurane or propofol anesthesia. Anesthesiology 2000;93(5):1205–9.
[43] Harper AM, Glass HI. Effect of alterations in the arterial carbon dioxide tension on the blood flow through the cerebral cortex at normal and low arterial blood pressures. J Neurol Neurosurg Psychiatr 1965;28(5):449–52.
[44] Ouchi T, Ochiai R, Takeda J, et al. Combined effects of propofol and mild hypothermia on cerebral metabolism and blood flow in rhesus monkey: a positron emission tomography study. J Anesth 2006;20(3):208–14.
[45] Maruyama M, Shimoji K, Ichikawa T, et al. The effects of extreme hemodilutions on the autoregulation of cerebral blood flow, electroencephalogram and cerebral metabolic rate of oxygen in the dog. Stroke 1985;16(4):675–9.
[46] Lee LA, Deem S, Glenny RW, et al. Effects of anemia and hypotension on porcine optic nerve blood flow and oxygen delivery. Anesthesiology 2008;108(5):864–72.
[47] Mizgala HF. The calcium channel blockers: pharmacology and clinical applications. Can Anaesth Soc J 1983;30(3 Pt 2):S5–10.
[48] Steen PA, Newberg LA, Milde JH, et al. Nimodipine improves cerebral blood flow and neurologic recovery after complete cerebral ischemia in the dog. J Cereb Blood Flow Metab 1983;3(1):38–43.
[49] Toni D, Frontoni M, Argentino C, et al. Update on calcium antagonists in cerebrovascular diseases. J Cardiovasc Pharmacol 1991;18(Suppl 8):S10–4.
[50] Sahlin C, Delgado T, Owman C, et al. Changes in cerebral blood flow and metabolism following intraarterial or local administration of nimodipine, before and after experimental subarachnoid hemorrhage in baboons. Stroke 1986;17(2):220–4.

[51] Alborch E, Salom JB, Torregrosa G. Calcium channels in cerebral arteries. Pharmacol Ther 1995;68(1):1–34.

[52] Frank Peacock W, Varon J, Ebrahimi R, et al. Clevidipine for severe hypertension in patients with renal dysfunction: a VELOCITY trial analysis. Blood Press Suppl 2011;1: 20–5.

[53] Szydlowska K, Tymianski M. Calcium, ischemia and excitotoxicity. Cell Calcium 2010;47(2):122–9.

[54] Marik PE, Varon J. Perioperative hypertension: a review of current and emerging therapeutic agents. J Clin Anesth 2009;21(3):220–9.

[55] Henriksen L, Thorshauge C, Harmsen A, et al. Controlled hypotension with sodium nitroprusside: effects on cerebral blood flow and cerebral venous blood gases in patients operated for cerebral aneurysms. Acta Anaesthesiol Scand 1983;27(1):62–7.

[56] Schoonman GG, van der Grond J, Kortmann C, et al. Migraine headache is not associated with cerebral or meningeal vasodilatation—a 3T magnetic resonance angiography study. Brain 2008;131(Pt 8):2192–200.

[57] Cottrell JE, Gupta B, Rappaport H, et al. Intracranial pressure during nitroglycerin-induced hypotension. J Neurosurg 1980;53(3):309–11.

[58] Hussain R, Tsuchida T, Kudo T, et al. Vasodilatory effect of adenosine triphosphate does not change cerebral blood flow: a PET study with (15)O-water. Ann Nucl Med 2009;23(8): 717–23.

[59] Rogers AT, Stump DA, Gravlee GP, et al. Response of cerebral blood flow to phenylephrine infusion during hypothermic cardiopulmonary bypass: influence of PaCO2 management. Anesthesiology 1988;69(4):547–51.

[60] Prielipp RC, Wall MH, Tobin JR, et al. Dexmedetomidine-induced sedation in volunteers decreases regional and global cerebral blood flow. Anesth Analg 2002;95(4):1052–9.

[61] Drummond JC, Dao AV, Roth DM, et al. Effect of dexmedetomidine on cerebral blood flow velocity, cerebral metabolic rate, and carbon dioxide response in normal humans. Anesthesiology 2008;108(2):225–32.

[62] Bryan RM Jr. Cerebral blood flow and energy metabolism during stress. Am J Phys 1990;259(2 Pt 2):H269–80.

[63] King BD, Sokoloff L, Wechsler RL. The effects of l-epinephrine and l-norepinephrine upon cerebral circulation and metabolism in man. J Clin Invest 1952;31(3):273–9.

[64] Ameredes BT. Beta-2-receptor regulation of immunomodulatory proteins in airway smooth muscle. Front Biosci (Schol Ed) 2011;3:643–54.

[65] Johansen JW, Schneider G, Windsor AM, et al. Esmolol potentiates reduction of minimum alveolar isoflurane concentration by alfentanil. Anesth Analg 1998;87(3):671–6.

[66] Johansen JW, Flaishon R, Sebel PS. Esmolol reduces anesthetic requirement for skin incision during propofol/nitrous oxide/morphine anesthesia. Anesthesiology 1997;86(2):364–71.

[67] Sassano-Higgins S, Friedlich P, Seri I. A meta-analysis of dopamine use in hypotensive preterm infants: blood pressure and cerebral hemodynamics. J Perinatol 2011;31(10): 647–55.

[68] Pfister D, Strebel SP, Steiner LA. Effects of catecholamines on cerebral blood vessels in patients with traumatic brain injury. Eur J Anaesthesiol Suppl 2008;42:98–103.

[69] Bandres J, Yao L, Nemoto EM, et al. Effects of dobutamine and dopamine on whole brain blood flow and metabolism in unanesthetized monkeys. J Neurosurg Anesthesiol 1992;4(4):250–6.

[70] Townsend JB, Ziedonis DM, Bryan RM, et al. Choroid plexus blood flow: evidence for dopaminergic influence. Brain Res 1984;290(1):165–9.

[71] Langsjo JW, Maksimow A, Salmi E, et al. S-ketamine anesthesia increases cerebral blood flow in excess of the metabolic needs in humans. Anesthesiology 2005;103(2):258–68.

[72] Algotsson L, Messeter K, Rosen I, et al. Effects of nitrous oxide on cerebral haemodynamics and metabolism during isoflurane anaesthesia in man. Acta Anaesthesiol Scand 1992;36(1):46–52.

[73] Laitio RM, Kaisti KK, Laangsjo JW, et al. Effects of xenon anesthesia on cerebral blood flow in humans: a positron emission tomography study. Anesthesiology 2007;106(6): 1128–33.
[74] McCullough AW. Some anomalies of the cerebral circle (of Willis) and related vessels. The Anatomical Record 1962;142:537–43.
[75] Macchi C, Catini C, Federico C, et al. Magnetic resonance angiographic evaluation of circulus arteriosus cerebri (circle of Willis): a morphologic study in 100 human healthy subjects. Ital J Anat Embryol 1996;101(2):115–23.
[76] Kapoor K, Singh B, Dewan LI. Variations in the configuration of the circle of Willis. Anat Sci Int 2008;83(2):96–106.
[77] Battacharji SK, Hutchinson EC, McCall AJ. The Circle of Willis—the incidence of developmental abnormalities in normal and infarcted brains. Brain 1967;90(4):747–58.
[78] van Raamt AF, Mali WP, van Laar PJ, et al. The fetal variant of the circle of Willis and its influence on the cerebral collateral circulation. Cerebrovasc Dis 2006;22(4):217–24.
[79] Drummond JC, Lee RR, Howell JP Jr. Case report: focal cerebral ischemia after surgery in the "beach chair" position: the role of a congenital variation of circle of Willis anatomy. Anesth Analg 2012;114(6):1301–4.
[80] Henderson RD, Eliasziw M, Fox AJ, et al. Angiographically defined collateral circulation and risk of stroke in patients with severe carotid artery stenosis. North American Symptomatic Carotid Endarterectomy Trial (NASCET) Group. Stroke 2000;31(1):128–32.
[81] Hoksbergen AW, Legemate DA, Csiba L, et al. Absent collateral function of the circle of Willis as risk factor for ischemic stroke. Cerebrovasc Dis 2003;16(3):191–8.
[82] Schomer DF, Marks MP, Steinberg GK, et al. The anatomy of the posterior communicating artery as a risk factor for ischemic cerebral infarction. N Engl J Med 1994;330(22):1565–70.
[83] Kameyama M, Okinaka SH. Collateral circulation of the brain with special reference to atherosclerosis of the major cervical and cerebral arteries. Neurology 1963;13:279–86.
[84] Carey BJ, Eames PJ, Blake MJ, et al. Dynamic cerebral autoregulation is unaffected by aging. Stroke 2000;31(12):2895–900.
[85] Carey BJ, Panerai RB, Potter JF. Effect of aging on dynamic cerebral autoregulation during head-up tilt. Stroke 2003;34(8):1871–5.
[86] Eames PJ, Blake MJ, Panerai RB, et al. Cerebral autoregulation indices are unimpaired by hypertension in middle aged and older people. Am J Hypertens 2003;16(9 Pt 1):746–53.
[87] Schmieder K, Moller F, Engelhardt M, et al. Dynamic cerebral autoregulation in patients with ruptured and unruptured aneurysms after induction of general anesthesia. Zentralbl Neurochir 2006;67(2):81–7.
[88] Meyer JS, Terayama Y, Takashima S. Cerebral circulation in the elderly. Cerebrovasc Brain Metab Rev 1993;5(2):122–46.
[89] Soul JS, Hammer PE, Tsuji M, et al. Fluctuating pressure-passivity is common in the cerebral circulation of sick premature infants. Pediatr Res 2007;61(4):467–73.
[90] Faraci FM, Baumbach GL, Heistad DD. Cerebral circulation: humoral regulation and effects of chronic hypertension. J Am Soc Nephrol 1990;1(1):53–7.
[91] Hoffman WE, Albrecht RF, Miletich DJ. Cerebrovascular and metabolic effects of SNP-induced hypotension in young and aged hypertensive rats. Anesthesiology 1982;56(6): 427–30.
[92] Nobili F, Rodriguez G, Marenco S, et al. Regional cerebral blood flow in chronic hypertension. A correlative study. Stroke 1993;24(8):1148–53.
[93] Collins R, Peto R, MacMahon S, et al. Blood pressure, stroke, and coronary heart disease. Part 2, Short-term reductions in blood pressure: overview of randomised drug trials in their epidemiological context. Lancet 1990;335(8693):827–38.
[94] Prevention of stroke by antihypertensive drug treatment in older persons with isolated systolic hypertension. Final results of the Systolic Hypertension in the Elderly Program (SHEP). SHEP Cooperative Research Group. JAMA 1991;265(24):3255–64.

[95] Strandgaard S, Paulson OB. Cerebral blood flow in untreated and treated hypertension. Neth J Med 1995;47(4):180–4.
[96] Shinyama H, Nagai H, Kawamura T, et al. Effects of long-term treatment with the calcium antagonist AE0047 on cerebrovascular autoregulation and hypertrophy in spontaneously hypertensive rats. J Cardiovasc Pharmacol 1997;30(5):616–22.
[97] Wong LJ, Kupferman JC, Prohovnik I, et al. Hypertension impairs vascular reactivity in the pediatric brain. Stroke 2011;42(7):1834–8.
[98] Chang YJ, Chang TC, Lee TH, et al. Predictors of carotid artery stenosis after radiotherapy for head and neck cancers. J Vasc Surg 2009;50(2):280–5.
[99] Tomura N, Otani T, Koga M, et al. Correlation between severity of carotid stenosis and vascular reserve measured by acetazolamide brain perfusion single photon emission computed tomography. J Stroke Cerebrovasc Dis 2011. [Epub ahead of print].
[100] Jongen LM, van der Worp HB, Waaijer A, et al. Interrelation between the degree of carotid stenosis, collateral circulation and cerebral perfusion. Cerebrovasc Dis 2010;30(3): 277–84.
[101] Bokkers RP, van Osch MJ, Klijn CJ, et al. Cerebrovascular reactivity within perfusion territories in patients with an internal carotid artery occlusion. J Neurol Neurosurg Psychiatr 2011;82(9):1011–6.
[102] Dalainas I, Avgerinos ED, Daskalopoulos ME, et al. The critical role of the external carotid artery in cerebral perfusion of patients with total occlusion of the internal carotid artery. Int Angiol 2012;31(1):16–21.
[103] Tang SC, Huang YW, Shieh JS, et al. Dynamic cerebral autoregulation in carotid stenosis before and after carotid stenting. J Vasc Surg 2008;48(1):88–92.
[104] Duan W, Chun-Qing Z, Zheng J, et al. Relief of carotid stenosis improves impaired cognition in a rat model of chronic cerebral hypoperfusion. Acta Neurobiol Exp 2011;71(2): 233–43.
[105] Brott TG, Hobson RW 2nd, Howard G, et al. Stenting versus endarterectomy for treatment of carotid-artery stenosis. N Engl J Med 2010;363(1):11–23.
[106] Furie KL, Kasner SE, Adams RJ, et al. Guidelines for the prevention of stroke in patients with stroke or transient ischemic attack: a guideline for healthcare professionals from the American Heart Association/American Stroke Association. Stroke 2011;42(1):227–76.
[107] van Mook WN, Rennenberg RJ, Schurink GW, et al. Cerebral hyperperfusion syndrome. Lancet Neurol 2005;4(12):877–88.
[108] Torgovnick J, Sethi N, Arsura E. Cerebral hyperperfusion syndrome occurring three weeks after carotid endarterectomy. Rev Bras Cir Cardiovasc 2007;22(1):116–8 [in English, Portuguese].
[109] Dalman JE, Beenakkers IC, Moll FL, et al. Transcranial Doppler monitoring during carotid endarterectomy helps to identify patients at risk of postoperative hyperperfusion. Eur J Vasc Endovasc Surg 1999;18(3):222–7.
[110] Coronado VG, Xu L, Basavaraju SV, et al. Surveillance for traumatic brain injury-related deaths—United States, 1997-2007. MMWR Surveill Summ 2011;60(5):1–32.
[111] Haubrich C, Steiner L, Kasprowicz M, et al. Short-term moderate hypocapnia augments detection of optimal cerebral perfusion pressure. J Neurotrauma 2011;28(7):1133–7.
[112] Budohoski KP, Czosnyka M, de Riva N, et al. The relationship between cerebral blood flow autoregulation and cerebrovascular pressure reactivity after traumatic brain injury. Neurosurgery 2012;71(3):652–61.
[113] Lewis PM, Smielewski P, Rosenfeld JV, et al. Assessment of cerebral autoregulation from respiratory oscillations in ventilated patients after traumatic brain injury. Acta Neurochir Suppl 2012;114:141–6.
[114] Beynon C, Kiening KL, Orakcioglu B, et al. Brain tissue oxygen monitoring and hyperoxic treatment in patients with traumatic brain injury. J Neurotrauma 2012;29(12):2109–23.
[115] Brady KM, Shaffner DH, Lee JK, et al. Continuous monitoring of cerebrovascular pressure reactivity after traumatic brain injury in children. Pediatrics 2009;124(6):e1205–12.

[116] Adelson PD, Srinivas R, Chang Y, et al. Cerebrovascular response in children following severe traumatic brain injury. Childs Nerv Syst 2011;27(9):1465–76.
[117] Pohl A, Cullen DJ. Cerebral ischemia during shoulder surgery in the upright position: a case series. J Clin Anesth 2005;17(6):463–9.
[118] Brondum E, Hasenkam JM, Secher NH, et al. Jugular venous pooling during lowering of the head affects blood pressure of the anesthetized giraffe. Am J Physiol Regul Integr Comp Physiol Oct 2009;297(4):R1058–65.
[119] McCulloch TJ, Liyanagama K, Petchell J. Relative hypotension in the beach-chair position: effects on middle cerebral artery blood velocity. Anaesth Intensive Care 2010;38(3): 486–91.
[120] Jeong H, Lee SH, Jan EA, et al. Haemodynamics and cerebral oxygenation during arthroscopic shoulder surgery in beach chair position under general anaesthesia. Acta Anaesthesiol Scand 2012;56(7):872–9.
[121] Sanford S. No day at the beach: catastrophic injuries in head-up position surgeries. Anesthesia the Law: A Risk Management Newsletter 2012;33:1–5.
[122] The Postoperative Visual Loss Study Group. Risk factors associated with ischemic optic neuropathy after spine surgery. Anesthesiology 2012;116(1):15–24.

Advances in Anesthesia 30 (2012) 131–146

ADVANCES IN ANESTHESIA

ELSEVIER MOSBY

Conversion to *ICD-10*

Implications for Anesthesiologists and Their Practices

Juhan Paiste, MD, MBA[a,b,*], Loretta Kowalick, RN, CMM[a], Maria D. Motovidlak-Thomas, CRNA, BA, MSN[c], Ivan J. Perry, DO[a,b]

[a]Allentown Anesthesia Associates, Inc, 1245 S. Cedar Crest Boulevard, Allentown, PA 18103, USA; [b]Department of Anesthesiology, Lehigh Valley Health Network, 1200 South Cedar Crest Boulevard, Allentown, PA 18103, USA; [c]Lehigh Valley Anesthesia Services, PC, 1200 South Cedar Crest Boulevard, Allentown, PA 18103, USA

Keywords

• *ICD-10* • International classifications • Anesthesiologists
• World Health Organization

Key Points

- The Centers for Medicare and Medicaid Services (CMS) should use the *International Classification of Diseases, Tenth Revision* (*ICD-10*) implementation delay to accelerate its efforts to incorporate the Systematized Nomenclature of Medicine—Clinical Terms (SNOMED CT) adoption and to ensure that all prerequisites and requirements to meet the new target conversion date are met on timely fashion.
- These measures include transaction testing between counterparties conducted on a clearly defined testing schedule—so that the industry will be ready on a new date. In the absence of guidance and oversight in these areas, it is possible that there once again will be calls for extensions as the new conversion date approaches.
- The Department of Health and Human Services (HHS) should prepare for the future by considering how the subsequent transition to the *ICD, Eleventh Revision* (*ICD-11*) can be gracefully accomplished. *ICD-11* is due for publication and adoption in approximately 2016.
- Physicians and practices are well advised to educate themselves and to prepare for a planned and controlled conversion to *ICD-10*, planning that will pay dividends regardless of the actual date for an eventual conversion.

INTRODUCTION

The World Health Organization (WHO) constitution mandates the production of international classifications on health so that there is a consensual, meaningful, and useful framework that governments, providers, and consumers can use as

*Corresponding author. *E-mail address*: Juhan.Paiste@lvhn.org

0737-6146/12/$ – see front matter
http://dx.doi.org/10.1016/j.aan.2012.06.001

a common language. Internationally endorsed classifications facilitate the storage, retrieval, analysis, and interpretation of data. They also permit the comparison of data within populations over time and between populations at the same point in time as well as the compilation of nationally consistent data.

The purpose of the WHO Family of International Classifications (WHO-FIC) is to promote the appropriate selection of classifications for the range of settings in the health field across the world. The WHO-FIC is comprised of reference classifications and derived classifications. Reference classifications are main classifications on basic parameters of health and consist of the (1) International Classification of Diseases (ICD), (2) International Classification of Functioning, Disability and Health, and (3) International Classification of Health Interventions [1].

The ICD is the international standard diagnostic classification that provides data code sets to define diseases, signs, symptoms, abnormal findings, complaints, social circumstances, and external causes of injury or disease. The ICD is published and copyrighted by the WHO (http://www.who. int/whosis/icd10/index.html) and is currently in its tenth revision [2].

HISTORY OVERVIEW

The development and continuing evolution of ICD reflects the untiring efforts of many people. Sir George Knibbs, the eminent Australian statistician, credited François Boissier de Lacroix (1706–1777), better known as Sauvages, with the first attempt to classify diseases systematically. Englishman William Farr (1807–1883), after the death of his wife from tuberculosis in 1838, joined the General Register Office of England and Wales and is credited with the collection of the first official medical statistics and causes of death in England and Wales [3].

The International Statistical Institute, the successor of the International Statistical Congress, during its meeting in Vienna in 1891, charged a committee chaired by Jacques Bertillon (1851–1922), Chief of Statistical Services of the City of Paris, with the preparation of a classification for causes of death. The report of this committee was presented by Bertillon at the meeting of the International Statistical Institute in Chicago in 1893 and was adopted. The classification prepared was based on the causes of death used by the City of Paris and represented a synthesis of English, German, and Swiss systems. It was based on the principle, adopted by William Farr, of distinguishing between general diseases and those localized to a particular organ or anatomic site. In 1898, the American Public Health Association, at its meeting in Ottawa, Canada, recommended the adoption of the Bertillon Classification by registrars of Canada, Mexico, and the United States.

In August 1900, the first International Conference for the Revision of the Bertillon, or International List of Causes of Death, was held in Paris. Delegates from 26 countries attended this conference and detailed the classification of causes of death into a comprehensive list of 179 groups and into a condensed classification of 35 groups. Adopted on August 21, 1900, this could be considered the birthdate of present-day ICD [4].

The dates of use for the first ICD and all revisions are as follows:

- *ICD-1* (1900–1909)
- *ICD-2* (1910–1920)
- *ICD-3* (1921–1929)
- *ICD-4* (1930–1938)
- *ICD-5* (1939–1948)
- *ICD-6* (1949–1957)
- *ICD-7* (1958–1967)
- *ICD-8*, adapted (1968–1978)
- *ICD-9* (1979–1998)
- *ICD-10* (1999–present)
- *ICD-11* (planned for 2016)

ICD-9 OVERVIEW

Since 2000, the United States has used the *ICD, Ninth Revision* (*ICD-9*), originally published in 1977, in the following forms: *ICD-9, Clinical Modification* (*ICD-9-CM*), used in all health care settings, and *ICD-9-Procedure Coding System* (*ICD-9-PCS*), used only for inpatient hospital settings [5].

The prevailing *ICD-9* classification has several limitations that prevent complete and precise coding and billing of health conditions and treatments, including

- Outdated terminology that is inconsistent with current medical practice
- Present code length and alphanumeric structure, limiting the number of new codes and many disease categories that are already full
- Codes lacking sufficient specificity and detail for
  - Accurate anatomic descriptions
  - Differentiation of risk and severity
  - Key parameters to differentiate disease manifestations
  - Optimal claim reimbursement
  - Value-based purchasing methodologies
- Lack of sufficient detail, which hinders the ability of payers and others to analyze information, such as health care use, costs and outcomes, resource usage and allocation, and performance measurement
- Existing codes that do not provide the level of detail necessary to further streamline automated claim processing, which would predictably result in fewer payer-physician inquiries, claim payment delays, and/or denials [6]

ICD-10 OVERVIEW

ICD-10 was developed in 1992 and designed to promote international comparability in the collection, processing, classification, and presentation of morbidity and mortality statistics, reimbursement systems, and automated decision support in medicine. Several developed countries (Australia in 1998, Canada in 2000, Germany in 2000, France in 2005, Sweden in 2007, and so forth) have implemented *ICD-10* for reimbursement and resource allocation in their health systems. The international version of *ICD-10* (ie, the original WHO edition) is used in approximately 110 countries, including the United

States, for mortality reporting and statistics [7]. *ICD-10* is copyrighted by the WHO, which owns and publishes the classification. WHO has authorized country-specific modifications to the *ICD-10*, however, providing they conform to WHO conventions, and several countries have undertaken modification of *ICD-10* (Australia, *ICD-10-AM*; Germany, *ICD-10-GM*, and so forth).

ICD-10 provides more specific data than *ICD-9* and better reflects current medical practice. *ICD-10* is a set of codes used to identify and describe diagnoses (*ICD-10-CM*) and procedures (*ICD-10-PCS*), replacing *ICD-9*, which has limited space available for new codes. *ICD-10* is more flexible and expands the number of codes in use from approximately 18,000 in the current *ICD-9* code set to approximately 140,000. Physicians will use *ICD-10-CM* to report diagnoses only and continue to report procedures with current procedural terminology (CPT) codes [8].

The added specificity and details within the *ICD-10* codes inform health care providers and health plans of patient incidence and history, which improves the effectiveness of case-management and care-coordination functions. Accurate coding also reduces the volume of claims rejected due to ambiguity. It is expected that *ICD-10* implementation will

- Improve operational processes across the health care industry by classifying detail within codes to accurately process payments and reimbursements
- Update the terminology and disease classifications to be consistent with current clinical practice and medical and technologic advances
- Increase flexibility for future updates as necessary
- Enhance coding accuracy and specificity to classify anatomic site, etiology, and severity
- Support refined reimbursement models to provide equitable payment for more complex conditions
- Streamline payment operations by allowing for greater automation and fewer payer-physician inquiries, decreasing delays and inappropriate denials
- Provide more detailed data to better analyze disease patterns and track and respond to public health outbreaks
- Provide opportunities to develop and implement new pricing and reimbursement structures, including fee schedules and hospital and ancillary pricing scenarios, based on greater diagnostic specificity
- Provide payers, program integrity contractors, and oversight agencies with opportunities for more effective detection and investigation of potential fraud or abuse, and proof of intentional fraud [9]

The National Center for Health Statistics, the federal agency responsible for the United States' use of WHO-FIC classifications, has developed the *ICD-10-CM*, a clinical modification of the classification for morbidity reporting purposes, to replace existing *ICD-9-CM* codes. The CMS have stated that all "covered entities"–as defined by the Health Insurance Portability and Accountability Act of 1996 (HIPAA)–are required to adopt *ICD-10* codes for use in all transactions governed by the HIPAA. The final rule adopting *ICD-10* as a standard was published in January 2009 and set a compliance date of October 1, 2013–a delay of 2 years from the compliance date initially specified in the 2008 proposed rule. On February 16, 2012, HHS Secretary Kathleen G. Sebelius announced that HHS would initiate a process to postpone the date by which certain health care entities must comply with *ICD-10* codes, and on April 9, 2012, a new target date was set for October 1, 2014 [10,11].

DIFFERENCES BETWEEN *ICD-9* AND *ICD-10*

The *ICD-9-CM* codes are only 3 to 5 digits long, and the alpha characters are limited to the letters V and E. The *ICD-10-CM* codes contain 3 to 7 alphanumeric characters. The greater number of digits and possible combinations allow identification of the body system, procedure, body part, laterality, approach, and any device involved in the surgery. The *ICD-10-CM* code set is more flexible for expansion and for the inclusion of new or added technologies and diagnoses.

Example of *ICD-10* code: S52.521A

S52—Fracture of forearm
S52.5—Fracture of lower end of radius
S52.52—Torus fracture of lower end of radius
S52.521—Torus fracture of lower end of right radius
S52.521A—Torus fracture of lower end of right radius, initial encounter for closed fracture
S52—States the category
S52.XY—4th and 5th Characters provide additional clinical detail and anatomic site
S52.XYZ—6th Character in this example indicates laterality ("right").
S52.XYZA—7th Character, "A," is an extension that provides additional information (initial encounter)

ICD-10 EFFECTS ON PHYSICIAN REIMBURSEMENTS

The transition to *ICD-10* will result in changes to most physician reimbursement models. The nature of these changes will vary based on each practice's individual contracting arrangements. Physician groups should include *ICD-10* in their payer contract negotiation discussions during the transition preparation and implementation process, to decrease the risk of compliance errors and claims denials. During the transition period after *ICD-10* implementation, payers will have little choice but to continue prior reimbursement policies. As implications of expanded, more detailed code sets become apparent, however, so too will the possibility for larger payments for greater complexity and smaller payments for lesser complexity.

Traditional CPT-based reimbursements will not be directly affected because these codes are not part of the *ICD-10* change. Decreases in cash flow may be anticipated, however, due to increased complexity of claims processing and reprocessing, staff learning curves, and changes in claims processing rules in payer systems as they attempt to adapt themselves into use of *ICD-10.* It may be advisable for practices or individual physicians to establish cash reserves for operational expenses or to consider obtaining a line of credit to cover cash flow disruptions.

For physician practices with contracts in capitated or case-based payments, significant impact can be anticipated because the reimbursement funds are defined differently in *ICD-10*. Reimbursements and risk adjustment models will be new, different, and untested. *ICD-10* will provide better insight into risk and severity over time but primarily if, and as, providers are able to capture accurate *ICD-10* data.

Comprehensive and detailed clinical documentation requirements will increase audit risk if documentation cannot support the new *ICD-10* detail. If audits reveal that payments were tied to inappropriate services based on *ICD-10*'s new definitions and rules, payers may require recovery of payments from providers.

The effect of *ICD-10* on evolving reimbursement models (such as episode and performance-based) and on accountable care organization models is still unclear. Because there are no historical data or benchmarks yet for *ICD-10*, there are poorly developed data for making episode-based or performance baselines for cost projections.

For performance-based and risk-sharing contracting arrangements, physician practices should keep in mind

- The complexity and risk of service based on severity of the conditions for which services are delivered, which could result in service-based payments adjusted either positively or negatively based on the complexity and risk assessment
- Complications, never events, preventable admissions, hospital-acquired conditions, patient safety, and other potentially avoidable detrimental patient impacts
- Outcomes as a consideration in the payment model based on a precise definition of a patient's condition and the institutional procedures to maintain or improve those conditions

TRANSITIONING FROM *ICD-9* TO *ICD-10*

The process of transition to new ICD coding will have a major impact on anyone who uses health care information that contains a diagnosis and/or inpatient procedure code, including

- Hospitals
- Health care practitioners and institutions
- Health insurers and other third-party payers
- Electronic transaction clearinghouses
- Hardware and software manufacturers and vendors
- Billing and practice management service providers
- Health care administrative and oversight agencies
- Public and private health care research institutions

To process *ICD-10* claims or other transactions, providers, payers, and vendors must first implement the Version 5010 electronic health care transaction standards mandated by HIPAA [12]. The existing HIPAA Version 4010 standards do not support the use of *ICD-10* codes. CMS set a deadline for Version 5010 transaction implementation for January 1, 2012, but has twice delayed enforcement–at the time of this writing until July 1, 2012 [13]. In his letter to CMS dated October 15, 2008, American Society of Anesthesiologists (ASA) president Dr Jeffrey Apfelbaum commented on the proposed *ICD-10* regulation, "ASA strongly believes that the implementation date for ICD-10 should be contingent on a successful conversion to Version 5010. We agree with others who have determined that a smooth and successful transition to ICD-10 will require a three year period that can start only once the 5010 conversion is complete" [14]. *Modern Healthcare*, on February 4, 2012, published an Emdeon vlearinghouse report stating compliance with 5010 standards currently stood at 65% for hospitals, physicians, and dentists, 55% for Medicaid, 70% for large commercial health plans, and 100% for Medicare [15].

ICD-9 VERSUS *ICD-10* VERSUS *ICD-11*? BENEFITS VERSUS CONSEQUENCES

Many larger hospital systems and medical groups have made significant investments in preparation to transition to *ICD-10* coding through redesigned computer programs, billing, and administrative training. Many smaller medical groups and hospitals, however, are not adequately prepared. On November 15, 2011, American Medical Association (AMA) President Peter W. Carmel stated, "The implementation of ICD-10 will create significant burdens on the practice of medicine with no direct benefit to individual patients' care. At a time when we are working to get the best value possible for our health care dollar, this massive and expensive undertaking will add administrative expense and create unnecessary workflow disruptions. The timing could not be worse as many physicians are working to implement electronic health records into their practices" [16].

Since the initiation of prospective payment and diagnosis-related groups in the early 1980s, the use of ICD coding in the United States has become tightly coupled with fee-for-service health care reimbursement. As a consequence, algorithms to project provider revenue, identify high-cost interventions, and improve the efficiency of health care delivery have evolved with an ICD-centered focus. The secondary uses of health information for purposes of quality management, clinical metrics, and research have likewise developed a strong dependence on ICD coding.

Although the CMS have estimated provider *ICD-10* adoption costs to be 0.03% of revenue, other conducted surveys suggest significantly higher costs [17]. Potential downstream disruptions, including quality metrics reporting, decision support systems, public health reporting, and research registries, will pose additional financial burdens for their users.

In a 2004 cost versus benefit analysis for HHS, the RAND Corporation offered an estimation of the costs and benefits associated with *ICD-10* implementation in the United States. The RAND report classified the associated costs into 3 categories:

- Costs of training
- Productivity losses
- System changes

The RAND Corporation report estimated cumulative total costs of *ICD-10* implementation over a 10-year period for training to be $200 to $480 million, productivity losses $50 to $400 million, and system changes $245 to $810 million. The majority of such costs will likely be borne by providers ($50 to $200 million) and commercial payers ($100 to $250 million).

To develop benefit estimates, the RAND Corporation developed a set of parameters based on plausible (but by no means inevitable) scenarios, to account for 5 major classes of benefits:

- More-accurate payments for new procedures
- Fewer miscoded, rejected, and improper reimbursement claims
- Better understanding of the value of new procedures
- Improved disease management
- Better understanding of health care outcomes (considered but not estimated)

Estimated benefits were calculated over a 10-year period and to come largely from the additional detail that *ICD-10-CM* and *ICD-10-PCS* offer. The RAND report emphasized, however, that to realize these benefits, providers must use the full codes, use them correctly, and use them in a fashion that is neutral to the reimbursement system. *ICD-9-CM* is by no means always completely, correctly, or neutrally exploited. The report suggested that erroneous, rejected, and questionable claims are likely to rise during predictable initial periods of confusion and that it may take 5 years to see positive cumulative benefits. These benefits, over a 10-year period, are estimated to fall in the range of $700 million to $7700 million, with a majority of the benefits coming from fewer rejected claims ($200 million to $2500 million), improved disease management ($200 million to $1500 million), and better understanding of new procedures ($100 million to $1500 million) [18,19].

It is reasonable to ask whether an increased number of codes, updated terminology, and additional specificity offered through *ICD-10* are sufficient justification for conversion. Proponents of *ICD-10* argue that its greater specificity and detailed coding options guard against fraud and abuse, increase clinical coding precision, and are more suitable for reimbursement and secondary uses alike.

Opponents to the conversion, however, have different views. Of *ICD-9-CM*'s 13,000 codes, approximately 65%, or approximately 8500 codes, describe different diseases, with the balance ascribed to injuries, health status, or services provided. In contrast, *ICD-10-CM* devotes only 30% of its 68,000 codes, or approximately 20,000 codes, to disease entities. Many of the new codes introduced in *ICD-10-CM* relate to identifying laterality or episode codes, such as first or subsequent treatment episode. Opponents argue that in reality, the difference between the 20,000 disease codes in *ICD-10-CM* and the 8500 in *ICD-9-CM* is an overestimate of the difference between the 2 versions of ICD. Opponents of *ICD-10* also point out that although *ICD-10* is an improvement over *ICD-9*, it is itself already 2 decades old, an outdated coding system drafted in the 1980s and published in 1990. Opponents argue that *ICD-10* coding does not reflect twenty-first century advances in health care. For example, *ICD-10* does not include any genomic information. As an example, if a woman undergoes a bilateral prophylactic mastectomy because of the presence of the BRCA2 gene (a genomic variant that increases the risk of breast cancer), there is no mechanism for coding this genomic variant as an indication for surgery.

Claims that *ICD-10* will do a much better job of coding clinical data, enabling more detailed and specific capturing of clinical events than its predecessor *ICD-9*, have been questioned. A study in Canada that examined dually coded administrative hospital discharge data, using both *ICD-9-CM* and *ICD-10-CM*, concluded that the functional capacity of *ICD-10-CM* was not materially different than that of *ICD-9-CM*. This means that in practical use, *ICD-10-CM* did not do a measurably better job of coding clinical data compared with *ICD-9* [20].

A full discussion of *ICD-10* implementation requires mention of the SNOMED CT. SNOMED CT is a systematically organized computer processable collection of medical terms providing codes, terms, synonyms, and definitions covering diseases, findings, procedures, microorganisms, substances, and so forth. It allows a consistent way to index, store, retrieve, and aggregate clinical data across specialties and sites of care. It helps organize the content of electronic health records systems, reducing the variability in the way data are captured, encoded, and used for clinical care of patients and research [21]. The Office of the National Coordinator for Health Information Technology has defined explicit stages, or levels, of electronic health record use that demonstrate the "meaningful use" of health information technology. Achieving these levels qualifies providers to receive financial incentives from CMS. During phase 1, the regulations recommend using SNOMED CT for clinical problems. Use of SNOMED CT clinical terminology is required under the phase 2 regulations for meaningful use, published on March 7, 2012 [22,23].

Meaningful use focuses on clinical activity and is independent of the reimbursement coding requirements of HIPAA. It is paramount that ICD coding systems work in concert with SNOMED CT. Although cross-mapping through data set crosswalks exists to translate between systems, it constitutes an enormous demand on payers' and providers' information technology resources. A requirement to simultaneously adopt *ICD-10* and SNOMED CT may impose an unsupportable burden on many providers and payers.

The *ICD-11* is under development by the WHO and its publication is expected in approximately 2016. *ICD-11* will be closely coupled to SNOMED CT, whose conceptual definitions and vocabulary was used to develop the description and logical architecture of *ICD-11*. Furthermore, *ICD-11* includes recent advances in medicine, including genomic content, and complements SNOMED CT in that *ICD-11* focuses on larger disease categories, whereas SNOMED-CT focuses on the highly detailed representation of a specific patient's conditions.

A memorandum of agreement and strong collaboration exist between the WHO and the International Health Terminology Standards Development

Organisation, which maintains SNOMED CT. This agreement includes commitments from each organization to maintain alignments between the systems, obviating future cross-mapping tools. *ICD-11* will be designed to include a foundation of defined and cross-linked disease and treatment information (mortality, morbidity, disability, quality indicators, and so forth); this interrelation is intended to allow query and study of several logically related but case-specific classifications, enabling data mining of relationships between cause, intervention, and outcome.

WILL *ICD-10* AND *ICD-11* IMPROVE PATIENT CARE?

Improved data may benefit the health care consumer and may assist in research efforts to determine if certain diseases are benefiting from specific treatments and interventions. Improved outcome information may enable patients to participate more meaningfully in the decision process of choosing treatment options.

ICD-10 and *ICD-11* may work to help satisfy the concerns of physicians in quality care, patient satisfaction, and reimbursement. Patient satisfaction may be enhanced if physicians involved in a patient's care collaborate more meaningfully to determine diagnosis and treatment. Bridging the communication gap among physicians should facilitate a quicker and better analysis of a patient's medical data, helping to avoid delays in diagnoses that may affect outcomes and increase health care costs. Better collaboration between providers would help decrease duplicity of testing, possibly shorten durations of hospitalizations for many patients, and contribute to cost savings, allowing greater capacity for insurance carriers to afford increased coverage for the growing health care needs of the population.

IMPLEMENTATION

To best achieve a smooth *ICD-10* transition, a practice should understand and consider the recommendations of CMS. These include

- Planning
- Communication and awareness
- Assessment
- Operational Implementation
- Testing
- Transition

During the planning phase, successful transition from *ICD-9* codes to *ICD-10* codes on October 1, 2014, will require significant resources [8]. It is important to establish a project management structure, governance, a plan to communicate with external partners, and risk management. Planning a comprehensive and realistic budget that includes costs, such as software upgrades and training needs, is essential. Contact vendors, physicians, affiliated hospitals, clearinghouses (electronic billing and claims services), and others to determine their plans for *ICD-10* transition [8]. Adhering to a well-defined timeline that makes sense for a practice will make the transition smoother [8].

Once the assessment of a practice's *ICD-10* transition needs is completed and the tasks required to complete this transition are planned, the next step is to determine what changes are needed to operations and systems to limit business risks and take advantage of opportunities.

Most physician practices depend on their vendors to provide support for the *ICD-10* transition. Vendors must first be verified, however, that they are prepared to meet the critical *ICD-10* transition needs and it should not be assumed that vendors will address the effects of the *ICD-10* implementation on key functional areas, including

- Patient registration
- Clinical documentation/health records
- Referrals and authorization
- Coding
- Order entry
- Billing
- Reporting and analysis
- Other diagnosis-related functions, depending on the nature of the practice

The potential impact of *ICD-10* to health care providers includes multiple system upgrades and testing cycles, increased human capital needs, significant training, increased claim denials, delayed and/or inaccurate payments, lost or reduced reimbursements and impacts to cash flow, and more complex financial reporting [9].

Although a practice may be well prepared, insurance carriers contract with may not be, and a backlog of reimbursements may be likely. Will state statutes requiring timely reimbursements for clean claims apply? If so, although interest may be paid on these outstanding claims, will there be enough resources to cover salaries, benefits, taxes, and so forth?

Both clinical and office personnel require time to familiarize themselves with the changes and to learn the new coding system. Because anesthesia charges involve multiple systems (ie, billing codes not only for the specialty of anesthesia but also for all interventional procedures associated with anesthesia care), learning will be more complex for billing personnel due to learning material encompassing all anatomic systems as thousands of additional diagnoses have been added. Charge entry personnel should begin learning these systems to understand the functionality of *ICD-10.* Resources are needed for educational training for both providers and office personnel in addition to upgrading software. Because everyone has a different learning curve, it may be beneficial to create a self-teaching program online through which personnel can access the learning material for review at home or at work in addition to the group teaching sessions. An online teaching tool allows personnel to learn and review at their own pace and at their own convenience. Software enhancements should be installed with adequate advance time for testing to ensure bugs in the system can be resolved.

Personnel need to be aware of the requirements and trained within a sufficient amount of time before *ICD-10* implementation to avoid confusion and delays in the operating systems of the practices. The American Association of Professional Coders provides a list of the 50 codes used most frequently in each system. This tool is useful to acquaint billing staff with how the current codes in *ICD-9* convert to codes in *ICD-10.* Billing personnel should be advised that *ICD-9* will also continue to be used for workers' compensation and disability claims.

If excellent communication between billing software personnel and insurance carriers is not optimal, now is the time to open those lines of communication. Ask questions and find out where the billing software company is in development. Keep in regular communication with representatives of insurance carriers and enquire what changes they will be making internally to both provider and patient health plans and if they are engaged in the process of transitioning to *ICD-10.* Understanding those changes and how they will have an impact the bottom line will help determine if a practice can continue participating with these health plans.

Make sure the software billing company can support both *ICD-9* and *ICD-10* because both will be used. Enquire when testing will be available. Testing several months before implementation is important to ensure how well the systems work together and allow for tweaking where necessary. Contact the ASA/AMA and investigate what tools are available for teaching. Encourage members of the billing staff to become certified as professional coders, who will likely then have a better understanding of the functionality of coding systems. Be prepared for insurance carriers to modify contract terms to comply with the specificity required in the *ICD-10* mandate as well as changes with coverage terms in patients' health plans that may require additional documentation to support patients' treatment plans. Providers will have to carefully consider all options of treatment available before prescribing tests or procedures, because they may be denied. Administrators may need to re-examine and perhaps renegotiate their contracts with insurance carriers.

Additional planning for the operational implementation phase of the *ICD-10* transition process should include the following key activities:

- Determine how the practice will work with vendors for implementation.
- Coordinate the update of the internal policies affected by *ICD-10* with the vendor.
- Coordinate the update of internal processes affected by *ICD-10*, including clinical, financial, actuarial, and reporting functions.
- Finalize system/technical requirements.
- Update approved code design to remediate system changes and updates.
- Coordinate update of code with vendor to remediate system changes/updates.
- Coordinate and conduct testing with partners based on updated system logic.
- Establish awareness among administrative and physician leadership involved in *ICD-10* implementation. This awareness should focus on the breadth of *ICD-10* impact across the health care industry and communicate a solid understanding of how this will affect business process, policy, and processes for the physician practice. Attention should be directed toward implementation costs, budget available, staff training needs, and affected vendor tools.

- Identify an *ICD-10* coordination manager who will create an inventory of key tasks for *ICD-10* implementation and be in charge of monitoring the daily activities associated with the *ICD-10* implementation, including
  - Developing an implementation plan and timeline
  - Conducting vendor evaluations, monitoring, and communication
  - Communication and awareness activities both internally and externally
  - Training needs assessment and identification
- Identify vendor support needs for the *ICD-10* implementation from vendors and health associations. In addition, identify other physician practices and agencies from which the practice may seek advice, assistance, or materials.

A formal implementation plan will be an important component for successful ICD-10 implementation. The suggested 9-steps for this approach are highlighted below, realizing that the size and complexity of a practice will determine the depth of investment in a formal plan.

9-Step implementation plan [24]

Inform

Give practice decision makers a high level overview of *ICD-10* and get buy-in to begin implementation preparation.

Assign

Assign individuals or teams to oversee the implementation effort, including available internal resources and any outsourced resources needed.

Assess

Assess all areas of practice and determine what has to change with an in-depth impact analysis, including documentation evaluations. Specificity is a key element of *ICD-10*.

Plan

Plan the implementation of *ICD-10*, including budgets, staff training, vendor communication, and policy and document changes with scheduled timetables.

Prepare

Prepare the changes for *ICD-10* by updating processes and policies and creating needed training materials. Begin changes with all vendors and outside partners.

Train

Train staff and providers on the changes made for *ICD-10*, including new policies and processes, code set training, software upgrades, anatomy and pathophysiology for *ICD-10*, and specificity requirements.

Test

Test all changes for *ICD-10* before implementation and verify at least 90% accuracy in documentation and coding.

Implement

Implement *ICD-10*.

Evaluate

Evaluate the implementation results, including review of denied claims, documentation, and coding accuracy. Analyze all changes and look for gaps between expectations and actual results to determine areas that need to have adjustments and then implement those changes.

It is crucial to use an implementation timeline to allow for the transition to *ICD-10.* Version 5010 needs to be implemented simultaneously if the organization has yet not done so [6]. A practice should

- Identify any additional tasks based on the practice's specific business processes, systems, and policies.
- Identify critical dependencies and predecessors.
- Identify resources and task owners.
- Estimate start and end dates.
- Identify entry and exit criteria between phases.
- Continue to update the plan throughout the *ICD-10* implementation and afterward.

SUMMARY

Christopher G. Chute (Chair, WHO *ICD-11* Revision Steering Group) concludes in a recent article that, "the ICD-10-CM conversion is expensive, arduous, disruptive, and of limited direct clinical benefit" [24]. Given, however, that *ICD-9* has simply run out of room for new codes and that there must be a replacement, as well as the reality that many payers, providers, and systems vendors have already invested heavily in *ICD-10* projects, the adoption of *ICD-10-CM*, there is significant momentum to proceed. Chute recommends "a delay period, with full adoption and use by all stakeholders by 2015" [25].

The authors of this review article agree with Chute that CMS should use the *ICD-10* implementation delay to accelerate its efforts to incorporate SNOMED CT adoption and to ensure that all prerequisites and requirements to meet the new target conversion date are met on timely fashion. These measures include transaction testing between counterparties, conducted on a clearly defined testing schedule–so that the industry is ready on a new date. In the absence of guidance and oversight in these areas, it is possible that once again there will be calls for extensions as the new conversion date approaches. Correspondingly, the HHS should prepare for the future by considering how the subsequent transition to *ICD-11* can be gracefully accomplished. *ICD-11* is due for publication and adoption in approximately 2016.

Unless and until such a delayed implementation decision is made, however, physicians and practices are well advised to educate themselves and to prepare for a planned and controlled conversion to *ICD-10*, planning for conversion to the new ICD will pay dividends regardless of the actual date for an eventual conversion.

References

[1] Madden R, Sykes C, Ustun T. World Health Organization family of International classifications: definition, scope and purpose. Available at: http://www.who.int/classifications/en/FamilyDocument2007.pdf. Accessed July 29, 2012.

[2] World Health Organization. International statistical classification of diseases and related health problems. 10th revision edition. World Health Organization; 2010 II.ICD-10. ISBN 978 92 4 154834 2. Available at: http://www.who.int/classifications/icd/ICD10Volume2_en_2010.pdf. Accessed July, 29, 2012.

[3] Moriyama IM, Loy RM, Robb-Smith AH. "History of the statistical classification of diseases and causes of death." March 2011 (DHHS publication; no. (PHS) 2011–1125) "March 2011." Available at: http://www.cdc.gov/nchs/data/misc/classification_diseases2011.pdf. Accessed July 29, 2012.

[4] World Health Organization. History of the development of the ICD. Available at: www.who.int/classifications/icd/en/HistoryOfICD.pdf. Accessed July 29, 2012.

[5] Steindel SJ. International classification of diseases, 10th edition, clinical modification and procedure coding system: descriptive overview of the next generation HIPAA code sets. J Am Med Inform Assoc 2010;17(3):274–82.

[6] Centers for Medicare, Medicaid Services Publication. "ICD-10 implementation guide for large practices". Available at: https://www.cms.gov/Medicare/Coding/ICD10/Downloads/ICD10LargePractices508-.pdf. Accessed July 29, 2012.

[7] Bowman S. Why ICD-10 is worth the trouble. J AHIMA 2008;79(3):24–9.

[8] Byrd J, Merrick S. Delayed or not: ASA will help you transition to ICD-10. ASA Newsletter 2008;72(10):20–2, 34. Available at: http://asatest.asahq.org/Newsletters/NL%20Portal/PDF/Oct08.pdf. Accessed July 29, 2012.

[9] Centers for Medicare, Medicaid Services Publication. "ICD-10 implementation guide for payers". Available at: www.cms.gov/Medicare/Coding/ICD10/Downloads/ICD10 Payers508.pdf. Accessed July 29, 2012.

[10] [Internet] Department of Health, Human Services. HHS announces intent to delay ICD-10 compliance date [press release]. Washington (DC): HHS; 2012. Available at: www.dhhs.gov/news/press/2012pres/02/20120216a.html. Accessed July 29, 2012.

[11] [Internet] Department of Health, Human Services. HHS proposes one-year delay of ICD-10 compliance [press release]. Washington (DC): HHS; 2012. Available at: http://www.hhs.gov/news/press/2012pres/02/20120216a.html. Accessed July 29, 2012.

[12] Leib M, Doyle CA, Merrick SK. Anesthesia claims and the 5010 Standard. ASA Newsletter 2012;76(3):42–3.

[13] "Extension of enforcement discretion period for updated HIPAA transaction standards through June 30, 2012". CMS statement March 15, 2012. Available at: www.cms.hhs.gov/Medicare/Coding/ICD10/Downloads/EnforcementDiscretionAnnouncement.pdf. Accessed July 29, 2012.

[14] ASA comment letter to CMS regarding ICD-10. October 15, 2008. Available at: http://www.asahq.org/For-the-Public-and-Media/Press-Room/News-Archives/~/link.aspx?_id=C9C2114E5B1045E19BD4AE8DE3860AF9&_z=z. Accessed July 29, 2012.

[15] Conn J. Rushing to comply. Providers, plans struggle to upgrade billing systems. Mod Healthc 2012;42(6):12. Available at: http://www.modernhealthcare.com/article/20120204/MAGAZINE/302049977#. Accessed July 29, 2012.

[16] Conn J. AMA opposes ICD-10. [serial on the Internet]. 2011 Nov 15 [cited 2012 Mar 14]. Available at: http://www.modernhealthcare.com/article/20111115/NEWS/311159956. Accessed July 29, 2012.

[17] Department of Health, Human Services. HIPAA administrative simplification: modifications to medical data code set standards to adopt ICD-10-CM and ICD-10-PCS. Fed Regist 2009;74(11):3328–62.

[18] Libicki M, Brahmakulam I. RAND Corporation report: The cost and benefit of moving to the ICD-10 code set, TR-132-DHHS. March 2004. Available at: www.rand.org/pubs/technical_reports/2004/RAND_TR132.pdf. Accessed July 29, 2012.

[19] Replacing ICD-9-CM with ICD-10-CM and ICD-10-PCS challenges, estimated costs, and potential benefits. Robert E. Nolan Company. Available at: http://www.renolan.com/healthcare/icd10study_1003.pdf. Accessed July 29, 2012.

[20] Quan H, Li B, Saunders LD, et al. Assessing validity of ICD-9-CM and ICD-10 administrative data in recording clinical conditions in a unique dually coded database. Health Serv Res 2008;43(4):1424–41.

[21] International Health Terminology Standards Development Organisation. SNOMED CT [home page on the Internet]. Copenhagen (Denmark): IHTSDO; 2012. Available at: http://www.ihtsdo.org/snomed-ct/. Accessed July 29, 2012.
[22] Department of Health, Human Services. Health information technology: standards, implementation specifications, and certification criteria for electronic health record technology, 2014 edition; revisions to the permanent certification program for health information technology. Fed Regist 2012;77(45):13832–85.
[23] Department of Health, Human Services. Health insurance reform; modifications to the Health Insurance Portability and Accountability Act (HIPAA) electronic transaction standards. Fed Regist 2009;74(11):3296–328.
[24] White Paper. ICD-10: The History, the Impact, and the Keys to Success AAPC Physician Services. http://www.rvpi.com/images/uploads/documents/ICD-10-white-paper-081511.pdf. Accessed July 29, 2012.
[25] Chute CG, Huff SM, Ferguson JA, et al. There are important reasons for delaying implementation of the new ICD-10 coding system. Health Aff 2012;31(4):836–42.

Advances in Anesthesia 30 (2012) 147–154

ELSEVIER
MOSBY

ADVANCES IN ANESTHESIA

Observational Data: Pitfalls and Pearls

Brian D. Sites, MD[a,b,*]

[a]Department of Anesthesiology, Dartmouth-Hitchcock Medical Center, One Medical Center Drive, Lebanon, NH, USA; [b]Department of Pain Management, Dartmouth-Hitchcock Medical Center, One Medical Center Drive, Lebanon, NH, USA

Keywords
• Hormonal replacement therapy • Observational research • Regression analysis
• Methodology

Key Points

- Observational research entails examining the relationship between exposures and outcomes. Cohort and case-control research methodologies are important in the context of rare outcomes and dangerous interventions, and for the external validation of randomized controlled trials.
- Observational research has the risk of drawing incorrect conclusions based on the presence of confounders.
- Regression analysis is the major technique for addressing potential confounders by providing adjusted estimates.

In medicine and anesthesiology, observational research is common and supports quality improvement, performance assessment, and clinical research. This article discusses the benefits and challenges of observational research.

OBSERVATIONAL DATA PROMISED SOMETHING SPECIAL

In the 1990s, it became clear that premenopausal women should take hormonal replacement therapy (HRT) as a preventive measure for many conditions such as dementia and coronary artery disease. After all, there were dozens of publications of observational data that were in full support of HRT [1–3]. The *Journal of the American Medical Association* (*JAMA*) went as far as constructing an elaborate prediction model that suggested an average woman taking HRT would extend her life by between 6 months and 3 years [4]. With respect to dementia prevention, the Cache County observational study followed more than 1800 women for a 3-year period and found that

*Department of Anesthesiology, Dartmouth-Hitchcock Medical Center, One Medical Center Drive, Lebanon, NH. *E-mail address*: brian.sites@hitchcock.org

0737-6146/12/$ – see front matter
http://dx.doi.org/10.1016/j.aan.2012.07.002

taking HRT resulted in a 44% reduction in the chance of experiencing dementia [5]. Journals were churning out supportive observational data at an impressive rate. Researchers even produced data demonstrating that HRT reduced mortality from all causes, including accidents and homicides [6]! Major medical professional organizations were recommending long-term use of HRT.

THEY WERE WRONG

By 2001, premarin sales had reached more than $2 billion [7]. There was one small problem, however. The proposed observational relationships between HRT and health benefits were wrong. In fact, asymptomatic women taking HRT were being subjected to increased risk. How do we know this? In 2002-2003, 2 key randomized controlled trials (RCTs), the Women's Health Initiative studies, were published in *JAMA* [8,9]. In the first study, 16,000 postmenopausal women were randomized to HRT or no HRT. After 5.2 years, HRT slightly reduced hip fractures and colon cancers, but increased the number of myocardial infarctions, cerebral vascular accidents, breast cancers, and thrombotic events. In the second study, 4500 postmenopausal women were enrolled and randomized to either HRT or no HRT. After 4 years of observation, 40 women receiving HRT had dementia and 21 women not undergoing HRT had dementia (relative risk = 2.05). The end result of these 2 huge trials was that millions of women were taken off the drug and the Food and Drug Administration slapped a black-box warning on premarin [10].

STUDY DESIGN

The gold standard for scientific research is the Randomized Controlled Trial (RCT). A RCT is attractive because the study groups can be considered to be identical in all ways measured and unmeasured. Thus, the interpretation of the difference after treatment will be due to the treatment rather than some other factor or factors. We will return to this "other factor" shortly. Under a RCT, the next quality level is observational data, which includes both cohort studies and case-controlled trials. The classic cohort study follows patients with and without an exposure and compares what happens to them over time. The Cache County trial is such an example. The idea was to recruit elderly women without dementia. The exposure was whether or not the women took HRT, and the outcome of interest was physician-diagnosed dementia. In contrast to prospective cohorts, case-control trials first start with identifying patients who have the outcome of interest. The control group is then formed by finding patients who are similar in every way to the cases except that they do not have the outcome. When the cases and controls are obtained, the researcher's primary objective is to see whether the exposure of interest is more common in the cases. Case-control trials are usually performed when the outcome of interest is rare.

METHODOLOGICAL PROBLEM: CONFOUNDING

The major problem with comparing 2 groups that were not randomly selected is that they may be distinctly different. Potential differences can exist in regard of a huge range of potential variables from socioeconomic characteristics to actual physical disease. In the HRT example, one can easily imagine that within the list of how the 2 groups are different may actually contain a third variable or variables having an impact on whether or not someone contracts dementia or coronary artery disease. In statistical language, this third variable is called a confounder. Confounding is considered the major impediment to drawing the correct conclusions from observational data. For a variable to be a confounder, it must be related to the proposed exposure and independently related to the outcome. Probably the most common confounder in medicine is age. As an example, Hospital A reports its mortality rate for craniotomy as 6% and Hospital B reports an 8% mortality rate. Which hospital should you go to when you need a craniotomy? The answer is that you don't know. It may very well be that Hospital A is better, but how would you interpret the results if you found out that Hospital A's average patient age is 47 and Hospital B's average age is 79 years? You would probably conclude that it is not "fair" to compare the mortality rates between the two hospitals because older patients are likely to have a higher perioperative mortality rate. In this example, age confounds the apparent relationship between exposure (Hospital A vs Hospital B) and the outcome, death.

TECHNIQUES TO COMPENSATE FOR CONFOUNDING

The fundamental objective of the research team in any observational data set is to try to statistically make the groups as similar as possible. Starting with study design, researchers will often restrict inclusion criteria to a certain type of patient. In a retrospective review of a large data set, this is often accomplished by limiting the analysis to only patients who have or do not have a certain medical condition or characteristic. For instance, if researchers are trying to examine the relationship between employment status and back pain, it would probably be prudent to exclude patients who were pregnant, thus effectively removing the possibility of this obvious confounder of back pain. After restriction, 2 common approaches are to adjust for the potential confounder or to simply provide strata-specific relationships. In the simple case of hospital exposure and mortality rates, the data can be adjusted for age by calculating what the mortality rate would be given the actual data if it were applied to a standard-age population; this is an example of direct age adjustment. A hospital that treats mostly young people will generate more failures (deaths) when applied to a standard population than a hospital that primarily treats older patients. Thus, when we interpret mortality rates adjusted for age, we are assessing the impact of the exposure (hospital) on the outcome (death) without the effect of age. Because older people are more likely to die, we must remove this classic confounder when assessing the relationship between hospital exposure and death. Arguably the simplest way to adjust for age (or another potential confounder) is to provide strata-specific results. For example:

Age (y)	Hospital A No. of deaths	No. treated	Mortality rate	Hospital B No. of deaths	No. treated	Mortality rate
<30	5	200	0.025	1	50	0.020
30–40	6	200	0.030	3	100	0.030
40–50	9	150	0.060	4	100	0.040
50–60	6	150	0.040	5	150	0.033
60–70	7	100	0.070	9	150	0.060
70–80	11	100	0.110	17	200	0.085
>80	13	50	0.260	41	200	0.205
Total	57	950	—	80	950	—
Crude rate	0.060			0.08		

In this example, even though the crude mortality rate is higher at Hospital B, you would be better off going here for your craniotomy if you are older than 40. Here, the age-specific mortality for Hospital B is better than that for Hospital A. Age is being used as an example of a classic confounder, but there are endless others. The major point is that researchers must think of, measure, and then adjust for confounders when analyzing observational data. This may seem like an easy task, but it is obvious from the results of the RCTs that the Cache County observational study missed some important confounders. There was something different about the patients who took HRT compared with those who did not, this despite collecting and adjusting for multiple variables in more than 1800 women.

STATISTICAL CONSIDERATIONS IN OBSERVATIONAL DATA

Exposures and outcomes can be organized into either continuous data or categorical data. Examples of continuous data would be blood pressure, hospital stay in days, and age. Categorical data can be dichotomous (yes/no), ordinal (American Society of Anesthesiologists [ASA] score), or simply nominal (surgery type). The various categories of ordinal data have value, but the interval values are not quantifiable. For example, an ASA III is healthier than an ASA IV, but the quantity of health between an ASA III and IV may not be the same as between an ASA I and II. Nominal data have no inherent value.

The explanation and use of various statistical tests to analyze observational data are beyond the scope of this review. Conceptually, however, the relationship between an exposure and outcome is usually examined first with standard univariate analysis. When outcome data are normally distributed and continuous, a Student *t*-test can be used with a dichotomous exposure. When outcome data are normally distributed and categorical, a χ^2 test can be applied to a categorical exposure. Usually the first step in assessing whether a variable may be acting as a confounder is to analyze its relationship with either the exposure or the outcome. This univariate analysis is the foundation for most "Table 1s" published in the literature.

The modern workhorse when analyzing observational data is regression analysis. Regression techniques allow the researcher to accomplish 3 major objectives: to measure the association when confounding is possible, calculate adjusted estimates, and predict outcomes. When the outcome is continuous, researchers use linear regression. When the outcome is dichotomous (eg, death), logistic regression is used. Regression analysis entails creating a mathematical model (based on the observed data) to predict an outcome.

A pertinent example of linear regression is the creation of a model predicting the miles per gallon (MPG) of a car based on 1 versus 2 variables. For this example we will use 1978 automobile data provided within the software STATA (StataCorp, College Station, TX). In this database, there is information on 74 different cars. Our outcome of interest is MPG. Using linear regression, we create a model that predicts MPG (outcome) as a function of price (exposure). Fig. 1 reveals this relationship. The individual data points are the cars and the superimposed line represents the best-fit line. This line is determined using the ordinary least squares (OLS) technique. The OLS technique minimizes the sum of the squared differences between the actual data points and the predicted value. The null hypothesis for a simple linear regression line is that the slope of the predicted line is zero. In this particular example, the slope of the line is −0.009. In statistical language, this value is known as the coefficient. The *P* value for the coefficient of price is <.001, meaning that we reject the null

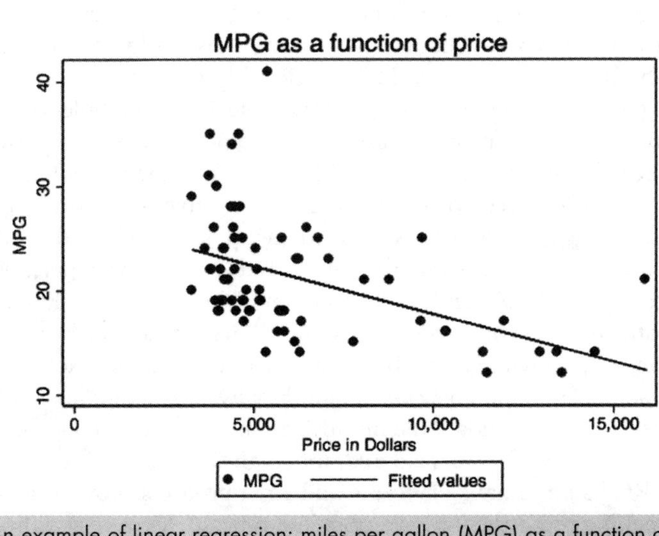

Fig. 1. An example of linear regression: miles per gallon (MPG) as a function of price.

hypothesis and can conclude that there is a statistically significant linear relationship between price and MPG. The coefficient can be interpreted as for every $1000 dollar increase in price; there is a loss of 0.9 MPG. It should be obvious that even though there appears to be a strong negative relationship between MPG and price, this apparent relationship is most likely confounded by a third (confounding) variable. Remember, for a variable to be considered a confounder, it must be related to the exposure (price) and independently related to the outcome (MPG). An obvious potential confounder is the weight of the car. As it turns out, heavier cars are more expensive, likely based on the added metal and so forth. In addition, heavy cars will obviously reduce MPG. When we formulate a linear regression model predicting MPG as a function of both weight and price, we now see that the coefficient for price is −0.0009, a factor of 10 less than when the model did not include weight. The *P* value has become nonsignificant at .56. Thus, price is not an independent predictor of MPG when we hold weight constant. It can be concluded that the apparent relationship of price to MPG is confounded by weight. Predicting an outcome by holding 1 or more variables constant to evaluate the independent effect of an exposure is a major function of a regression model. One can see that the original relationship in Fig. 1 is not accurate. When the confounding effect of weight is taken into account, the relationship between MPG and price is not linear.

WHY EVER PERFORM OBSERVATIONAL RESEARCH?

There are several situations in which observational data are necessary because RCTs cannot or should not be performed. First, RCTs should not be done when there is known harm from getting or not getting the treatment. For instance, Surgenor and colleagues [11] examined the risk of intraoperative blood transfusion during coronary artery bypass grafting and mortality. The data were gathered from a multistate clinical registry in which patients getting 1 to 2 packed red blood cells had a 1.67-times risk of death compared with patients who did not get blood. This relationship existed even after adjusting (controlling for) many potential cofounders such as multiple comorbidities and ejection fraction. This exposure and outcome represents a perfect match for an observational analysis, as it would be hard to imagine an RCT in which patients were randomized to receive or not to receive a transfusion based on controversial triggers. Second, RCTs are not helpful when the outcome is rare. For instance, if we assume the rate of nerve injury is 1 per 3000 blocks with an α value of .05 and a β value of .90, it would take more than 200,000 patients per group to demonstrate a 50% reduction in a new nerve-block technique. Obviously such a study would be impossible, both from a practical standpoint and cost standpoint. Finally, a great indication for observational research is to validate the findings of an RCT. This concept may seem odd, in that an RCT is considered the highest level of clinical research. However, RCTs often have elaborate and strict protocols governing treatment delivery, making reproduction on a population-health level very difficult. Thus, RCTs may lack external validity. Observational research can place conceptual issues learned from RCTs into real-world scenarios. For instance, Goodney and colleagues [12] analyzed a clinical registry of the Vascular Study Group of New England for potential cardiac morbidity reduction related to an increasing use of perioperative β-blocker medications. Despite an increase in perioperative β-blocker treatment from 68% to 88% by the participating centers, there was no statistical change in the rate of postoperative myocardial infarction. This finding stands in contrast to the multiple RCTs supporting the reduction in morbidity associated with β-blocker administration. A likely reason for this difference is that the real-world administration of β-blockers was not goal directed and dose standardized as it typically is in RCT protocols.

SUMMARY

Observational research entails examining the relationship between exposures and outcomes. Cohort and case-control research methodologies are important in the context of rare outcomes and dangerous interventions, and for the external validation of RCTs. Observational research has the risk of drawing incorrect conclusions based on the presence of confounders. Regression analysis is the major technique for addressing potential confounders by providing adjusted estimates.

Acknowledgments

The author would like to acknowledge the teaching and education provided by Dr Gilbert Welch, M.D., M.P.H from the Dartmouth Institute. The age adjustment example was modified with approval from Dr Welch's curriculum.

References

[1] Stampfer M, Colditz G. Estrogen replacement therapy and coronary heart disease: a quantitative assessment of the epidemiologic evidence. Prev Med 1991;20:47–63.
[2] Bush TL, Barrett-Connor E, Cowan LD, et al. Cardiovascular mortality and noncontraceptive use of estrogen in women: results from the Lipid Research Clinics Program follow-up study. Circulation 1987;75:1102–9.
[3] Grady D, Rueben SB, Petitti DB, et al. Hormone therapy to prevent disease and prolong life in postmenopausal women. Ann Intern Med 1992;117:1016–37.
[4] Col NF, Eckmen MH, Keris R, et al. Patient-specific decisions about hormone replacement therapy in premenopausal women. JAMA 1997;277:1146–7.
[5] Zandi PP, Carlson MC, Plassman BL, et al. Hormone replacement therapy and incidence of Alzheimer disease in older women the cache county study. JAMA 2002;288:2123–9.
[6] Petitti DB, Perlman JA, Sidney S. Postmenopausal estrogen use and heart disease. N Engl J Med 1986;15:131–6.
[7] Available at: http://www.nytimes.com/2002/07/10/us/wyeth-stock-falls-24-after-report.html. Accessed February 14, 2012.
[8] Rossouw JE, Anderson GL, Prentice RL, et al. Risks and benefits of estrogen plus progestin in healthy postmenopausal women: principal results from the Women's Health Initiative randomized controlled trial. writing group for the women's health initiative investigators. JAMA 2002;288:321–33.
[9] Shumaker SA, Legault C, Rapp SR, et al. Estrogen plus progestin and the incidence of dementia and mild cognitive impairment in postmenopausal women: the Women's Health Initiative Memory Study: a randomized controlled trial. JAMA 2003;289:2651–62.

[10] FDA information. Available at: http://www.fda.gov/Safety/MedWatch/SafetyInformation/SafetyAlertsforHumanMedicalProducts/ucm153355.html. Accessed February 14, 2012.
[11] Surgenor SD, Kramer RS, Olmstead EM, et al. The association of perioperative red blood cell transfusions and decreased long-term survival after cardiac surgery. Anesth Analg 2009;108:1741–6.
[12] Goodney PP, Jorgensen JE, Nolan BW, et al. A regional quality improvement effort to increase beta-blocker administration before vascular surgery. J Vasc Surg 2011;53(1316):1328.

Advances in Anesthesia 30 (2012) 155–169

ADVANCES IN ANESTHESIA

Checklists, Briefings, and Operating Room Safety

Michael F. Mulroy, MD

Department of Anesthesiology, Virginia Mason Medical Center, 1100 Ninth Avenue, Seattle, WA 98101, USA

Keywords
• Checklists • Briefings • Patient safety

Key Points

- Preoperative checklists have been shown to be highly effective in improving compliance with safety steps and reducing perioperative morbidity and mortality.
- Their effectiveness seems to be enhanced when they are used as a framework for a team briefing that is used to improve communication and promote team behaviors, including empowering junior staff to question more senior authority figures and feeling free to communicate their concerns.
- It seems such a cultural change is essential to ensure full implementation and sustainability of a preprocedural pause/checklist and to effect significant improvements in patient safety.
- There also seems to be an increasing role for these cognitive aids in assisting physicians in handling evidence-based pathways and emergency situations.

INTRODUCTION

Mistakes happen. The inevitability of human error has been the subject of an entire discipline of science, documenting the mechanisms by which fallible humans are doomed to error, from simply losing car keys to miscalculating a dose of critical medications. Limited memory span (the number of objects an average human can hold in working memory is 7 ± 2, frequently referred to as "Miller's Law") and variable attention span (susceptible to multiple distractions and fatigue) make mistakes unavoidable in daily life and the workplace. Theorists have devised multiple approaches and tools to reduce the frequency of errors, particularly to avoid having multiple errors accumulate to produce a significant adverse outcome [1]. The major shift in recent approaches to error prevention is to move away from "blaming" individuals (who are usually trying

No funding support was received for this article.

E-mail address: Michael.Mulroy@vmmc.org

0737-6146/12/$ – see front matter
http://dx.doi.org/10.1016/j.aan.2012.07.004

very hard) to identifying the "systems" barriers to avoiding error. Multiple cognitive aids and thought-structuring tools have been developed [2]. This article focuses on the most elementary, the development of a checklist. A checklist roughly defined is a list of "to do" items, from as simple as a grocery list to as complex as the steps needed for a moon landing. Recent large-scale catastrophes, such as the airplane disaster on Tenerife and the Chernobyl nuclear power plant accident, have emphasized the need for adoption of more and more stringent tools to reduce human error.

HISTORY OF THE CHECKLIST

The first significant industrial checklist was developed in the aviation industry. In 1934, Boeing Aircraft Company was submitting a proposed heavy bomber to the Army Air Corps in the hopes of obtaining a large order. Although the plane had performed extremely well in initial trials, on the day of the final phase of evaluations, an army pilot took off in a test model and crashed the plane shortly after becoming airborne. Subsequent review showed that the test pilot was unfamiliar with the controls and had failed to release the elevator lock before take off. Boeing was subsequently given a very limited order for 13 planes. The pilots assigned to this new squadron recognized that this new model was a complex aircraft that may be "too much for one man to fly." The pilots developed a new tool to make sure that everything was done for the flight and that nothing was overlooked; it was a checklist. They actually developed four checklists (take off, flight, landing, and after landing). Their squadron subsequently flew 1,800,000 miles without an accident and the army eventually ordered 12,731 of the B-17 bombers [3]. Since that time, military and commercial aviation has relied extensively on a series of checklists for their normal operative procedures and for all emergency procedures. The ultimate vindication and a public embrace of this type of "cognitive aide" may have occurred when the crew of the US Airways flight out of LaGuardia in January 2009 was able to perform an emergency landing in the Hudson River and save all 155 persons aboard despite the loss of both engines. Coincidentally, within 2 weeks of that highly publicized, heroic event, *The New England Journal of Medicine* published a monumental report about the success of the use of a presurgical checklist to reduce mortality and morbidity in surgical procedures in eight study hospitals around the world [4].

TYPES OF CHECKLISTS

There are many forms of checklists, although all are designed to provide a standardization of a task and to remove the reliance on (fallible) human memory. Simple mnemonics are best known to medical students. Others are lists of tasks to be done in order, a "read-do" format. More complex forms include "read-do-verify," such as pilots do before take-off. When a group is involved, the format can expand to "verify and confirm," as would be most appropriate in the operating room (OR) [5]. Checklists can also be available for emergency situations, not just routine events, such as the ones used in the Hudson river plane landing. Although other industries have developed formal systems for constructing, testing, and revising checklists [6], medicine has been slow to embrace a pattern for checklist development [7].

CHECKLISTS AND THE MEDICAL COMMUNITY

The development of medical checklists has lagged significantly behind other high-risk and high-reliability industries, such as aviation and nuclear power. Many factors may contribute to lag. One of the primary reasons may be the reliance of the medical professional on individual "perfection" in an industry that has remained basically a one-on-one service for centuries [8]. This reliance on individual performance may well have been appropriate at a time when there were few drugs available and even less knowledge of medical illnesses, but the rapid development of scientific knowledge starting in the middle of the twentieth century has made it almost impossible for individuals to practice the highest level of care in every instance. Although the medical industry (perhaps because of its solo practice model) never experienced the catastrophic publicity of Tenerife or Chernobyl, the cumulative effect of multiple individual errors was brought to light by the Institute of Medicine report "To Err is Human" in 1999 [9]. That report suggested, based on cumulative information from several studies of medical errors, that somewhere between 44,000 and 98,000 patients died each year in the United States because of medical errors. The report stimulated a movement toward programs designed to improve patient safety and outcome, including standardization of processes, adoption of evidence-based medicine, and the development of more cognitive aids to assist the medical profession in rising to a level similar to other high-reliability industries. The Institute of Medicine report itself commented on the use of checklists in other industries as a tool to avoid errors, a concept that was already introduced by Leape [8] in his earlier 1994 essay on error in medicine. Others also recommended adopting "systems" approaches to improved team performance and error reduction, such as the airline industry's standard procedures and checklists [10,11]. Nevertheless, progress was slow, in part related to the traditional solo perfectionist pattern of medical practice and the long tradition of physician autonomy.

EARLY MEDICAL CHECKLISTS

Still, there were models of checklist use in medicine. The earliest checklist in medicine was the use of a "read-do" checklist for the anesthesia machine. This was primarily an equipment issue rather than clinical care, but it was a topic readily suitable for the checklist format. Because of data that showed complications related to equipment malfunction, various forms of a checklist were created, modified, and circulated. In 1986, the American Society of Anesthesiologists published in conjunction with the US Food and Drug Administration a generic checklist, the Anesthesia Apparatus Checklist. Although not perfect in detecting all errors [12], this checklist has been credited with a significant increase in safety. A study from the Netherlands in 2005 showed use of the checklist yielded a 0.64 odds reduction of morbidity or mortality compared with not using the checklist [13].

Checklists were also found to be useful to assist in adopting clinical pathways. Wolff and colleagues [14] reported that the inclusion of checklists between 1999 and 2002 significantly increased compliance with their medical pathways for treatment of acute myocardial infarction and stroke. Although compliance did not reach 100% with all parameters, it increased between 20% and 40% for each element of the acute myocardial infarction bundle, and was sustained for the 2-year study period. Other simple checklists have been used to assist clinicians in the diagnosis of brain death [15], management of diabetes [16], and end-of-life care in the intensive care unit (ICU) [17].

One of the major initial initiatives to spread the use of medical checklists came from the ICU group at The Johns Hopkins Medical Center. They found ambiguity and lack of clarity on their daily rounding, which they approached with a daily rounding goal sheet in 2003 [18]. The team at Johns Hopkins found that critical steps in patient progress were frequently missed in the complex atmosphere of the critical care unit, and that treatments and discharge were sometimes delayed because of lapses in communication. They created an outline of the daily report that included specific questions about steps in patient progress, and that each team, including physicians and nurses, was required to follow at the beginning of the day. They found that use of this simple tool reduced the length of stay of the average patient from 2.2 to 1.1 days.

This same group also focused their attention on a specific ICU complication: central line–associated blood-borne infections. Catheter related bloodstream infections (CRBSI) were known to be a serious risk to patients, but they persisted despite several known strategies for prevention (hand washing, use of mask and gown, full body barriers, chlorhexidine skin preparation, avoidance of the groin, sterile dressing, and early removal [19]). Although infections were not perceived as overly frequent, the current incidence of two to five infections per 1000 catheter days in any given ICU would produce a national total of 80,000 annual infections and 28,000 deaths, at an estimated cost of $2.3 billion. The Hopkins team implemented all of the known preventive measures coupled with a mandatory contemporaneous read-confirm checklist for insertion of all central lines, with an associated empowerment of the nursing staff to "stop the line" if the providers at any time were deviating from the checklist [20]. This process was tested between 1998 and 2002, and produced a reduction of CRBSI from 11.3 per 1000 catheter-days to zero.

After the success of this intervention, the team from Johns Hopkins was invited by the Agency for Healthcare Research and Quality to participate in a larger trial involving all of the ICUs in the state of Michigan. A total of 103 units participated between October 2003 and March 2005 in implementing the "Central Line Bundle," including the use of the checklist. They also implemented the daily goal process, steps to reduce ventilator-associated pneumonia, and other safety steps, but the Agency for Healthcare Research and Quality study focused on CRBSI. The median rate fell from 2.7 infections per 1000 catheter days to zero after 3 months. The mean rate also fell from 7.7 to 1.4 infections per 1000 catheter-days at the conclusion of the study at 18 months [21]. Since publication of these results, this "Central Line Bundle" has become a standard of care in the United States. It is an example of how a checklist can enhance the performance of evidence-based care.

APPLYING CHECKLISTS TO SURGERY

Although this ICU experience showed significant improvements in patient care, the OR remained a major source of patient morbidity and mortality. Several groups in North America approached the issue of surgical safety, usually starting from the perspective of improved communications, stimulated by the Joint Commission's emphasis on assessment of communication and "hospital culture" in 2007. Several institutions set out to improve team communications, usually through a preoperative briefing centered on a checklist.

One of the first reports was a preoperative briefing project initiated in the Kaiser Permanente hospital system in southern California. This group used a variation of the Safety Attitudes Questionnaire (SAQ) (developed for the airline industry) to assess teamwork and safety attitudes among their surgical staff. A multidisciplinary OR team then developed a preoperative briefing protocol that included team introductions and review of the surgical plan. After introduction of this format in 2002, they found significant improvements in their teamwork scores and elimination of wrong-site surgery in their hospitals in the reporting period [22].

The Johns Hopkins group that had studied the ICU experience also developed a briefing tool for surgery (Fig. 1), prompted by another Joint Commission mandate for a "Universal Protocol for Preventing Wrong Site, Wrong Procedure, Wrong Person Surgery" in 2004 [23]. The Hopkins team initiated their briefings in 2005, and also measured teamwork attitudes with a variant of the SAQ that included an assessment of the teams' perception of the risk of wrong-site events. Their tool significantly reduced the perceived risk of wrong-site events [24] and reduced OR delays [25].

In Canada, an in-depth approach to team communications followed the initial idea of a systems-based approach to error reduction [10]. Lingard and coworkers [26] studied OR communication patterns extensively, and identified several patterns of communication failures that increased the potential for error. They then developed a checklist to serve as a template for communication in the preprocedural briefing in 2003. Using this tool, they observed a decrease in communication errors from 3.95 per procedure to 1.31, with 34% of the briefings associated with "clinical utility" in terms of identifying problems and resolving knowledge gaps [27]. Further study showed this briefing was associated with increased compliance with preoperative antibiotic administration [28].

THE WORLD HEALTH ORGANIZATION SAFE SURGERY PROJECT

The World Health Organization (WHO) Safe Surgery Saves Lives Project eventually provided the major impetus for the widespread adoption of preprocedural checklists in the OR in 2008. This started with the publication of the guidelines

- ☐ **Introduction of first names and roles which are written on the whiteboard**
- ☐ **Review critical information**
  - ☐ Do we have the correct patient?
  - ☐ Is the correct side or site marked?
  - ☐ Has the procedure been agreed upon?
  - ☐ Have antibiotics been given?
- ☐ **Identify and Mitigate Hazards**
- ☐ **SURGERY:** Discuss plans for the surgical procedure:
  - ☐ Describe critical steps
  - ☐ Provide team with pertinent information, including problems that may be encountered
  - ☐ Ask team: If something were to go wrong with this procedure, what would it be, and how could we prevent the problem?
  - ☐ Risks during procedure, such as bleeding, fluid loss
  - ☐ Surgeon suggests, "If anyone has a concern during the case, please let me know."
- ☐ **ANESTHESIOLOGY:** Discuss all relevant issues:
  - ☐ Patient co-morbid disease that will increase risk
  - ☐ Aspects of surgery that increase risk, such as need for IV access
  - ☐ Availability of blood products
  - ☐ Interventions to prevent complication, such as myocardial infarction, surgical site infection
- ☐ **NURSING:** Discuss all relevant issues:
  - ☐ Are all necessary instruments available?
  - ☐ Will any special equipment be considered?
  - ☐ Plan for breaks (relieving nurse to introduce himself or herself when switching)

Fig. 1. Operating room briefing checklist. (*From* Makary MA, Mukherjee A, Sexton JB, et al. Operating room briefings and wrong-site surgery. J Am Coll Surg 2007;204:236–43; with permission.)

identifying multiple recommended practices to ensure surgical patients' safety worldwide [29]. Based on these guidelines, a working group was formed to design a 19-item checklist intended to be used globally to reduce the rate of complications (Fig. 2) [30]. This checklist was developed using technical advice from aviation experts in the design of checklists [6,10,31] and using an iterative process among panel members representing hospitals in the eight countries in which the checklist would be implemented and studied. The three-part document was designed to be used before induction of anesthesia, immediately before incision, and before the patient left the OR. A complex intervention was initiated in eight countries (Jordan, India, United States, Tanzania, Philippines, Canada, England, and New Zealand) including hospitals of various sizes, economic background, and presumed levels of medical sophistication. The intervention consisted of a pretrial observation period followed by the implementation of the use of a WHO checklist for nonemergent noncardiac adult surgeries, coupled with mandatory inclusion of monitoring with pulse oximetry, antibiotic coverage, and a preprocedural briefing by the surgical team. After

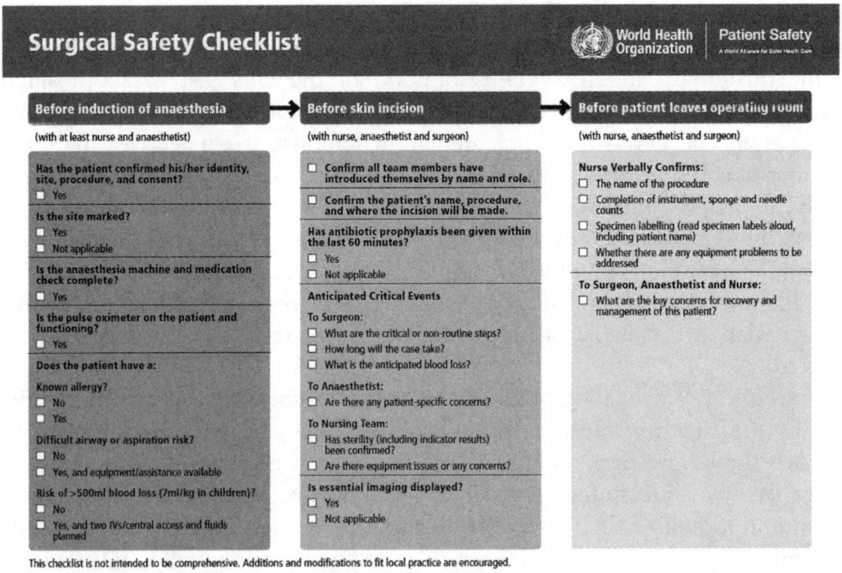

Surgical Safety Checklist

World Health Organization | Patient Safety

Before induction of anaesthesia → **Before skin incision** → **Before patient leaves operating room**

Before induction of anaesthesia

(with at least nurse and anaesthetist)

Has the patient confirmed his/her identity, site, procedure, and consent?
- ☐ Yes

Is the site marked?
- ☐ Yes
- ☐ Not applicable

Is the anaesthesia machine and medication check complete?
- ☐ Yes

Is the pulse oximeter on the patient and functioning?
- ☐ Yes

Does the patient have a:

Known allergy?
- ☐ No
- ☐ Yes

Difficult airway or aspiration risk?
- ☐ No
- ☐ Yes, and equipment/assistance available

Risk of >500ml blood loss (7ml/kg in children)?
- ☐ No
- ☐ Yes, and two IVs/central access and fluids planned

Before skin incision

(with nurse, anaesthetist and surgeon)

- ☐ **Confirm all team members have introduced themselves by name and role.**
- ☐ **Confirm the patient's name, procedure, and where the incision will be made.**

Has antibiotic prophylaxis been given within the last 60 minutes?
- ☐ Yes
- ☐ Not applicable

Anticipated Critical Events

To Surgeon:
- ☐ What are the critical or non-routine steps?
- ☐ How long will the case take?
- ☐ What is the anticipated blood loss?

To Anaesthetist:
- ☐ Are there any patient-specific concerns?

To Nursing Team:
- ☐ Has sterility (including indicator results) been confirmed?
- ☐ Are there equipment issues or any concerns?

Is essential imaging displayed?
- ☐ Yes
- ☐ Not applicable

Before patient leaves operating room

(with nurse, anaesthetist and surgeon)

Nurse Verbally Confirms:
- ☐ The name of the procedure
- ☐ Completion of instrument, sponge and needle counts
- ☐ Specimen labelling (read specimen labels aloud, including patient name)
- ☐ Whether there are any equipment problems to be addressed

To Surgeon, Anaesthetist and Nurse:
- ☐ What are the key concerns for recovery and management of this patient?

This checklist is not intended to be comprehensive. Additions and modifications to fit local practice are encouraged.

Fig. 2. World Health Organization surgical safety checklist (first edition). (*From* World Health Organization. Surgical safety checklist. Available at: http://www.who.int/patientsafety/safesurgery/ss_checklist/en/index.html.)

implementation, 3955 patients were followed for outcomes and complications. The rate of any complication across all of the sites dropped from 11% at baseline to 7% after use of the checklist. The total in-hospital death rate dropped from 1.5% to 0.8%, a statistically significant improvement [32]. Unplanned reoperations and surgical site infections also dropped. The changes were equally prevalent among the high-income and low-income sites, although the change in death rate was not significant in the high-income sites. The performance of the designated six safety steps associated with the protocol also increased significantly in the postimplementation period. A parallel investigation of urgent surgical procedures in the same hospitals using a similar protocol also showed a reduction in morbidity (from 18.4% to 11.7%) and mortality (from 3.7% to 1.4%), further supporting use of the pause and the checklist [33].

After publication of this study in January 2009, there was a groundswell of support for the use of preprocedural checklists, encouraged by the WHO itself and by the Joint Commission in the United States. The WHO reported that as of April 2010, 3791 hospitals in 120 countries had registered in the Safe Surgery Saves Lives program, which included implementation of the checklist. Twenty-five separate nations had mobilized resources to implement the WHO surgical safety checklist at a national level [34]. In the United States, the State of Washington (which was home to one of the original eight study sites) instituted adoption of the checklist in all hospitals in the state by March 2010.

INITIAL SUCCESS OF THE WHO CHECKLIST

The advantageous effects of the use of the checklist were confirmed by a report from Amsterdam in 2012 [35]. Adoption of the checklist in six hospitals, compared with a 3-month observation period before use of the checklist, in 3820 patients observed after implementation demonstrated a decrease in the total number of complications from 27.3% to 16.7%. In that group, as in the original study, in-hospital mortality decreased from 1.5% to 0.8%. Outcomes did not change in a group of control hospitals in the same area during the same time period. The hospitals involved in this study were all perceived to be functioning at a "high standard of care" before the intervention, confirming that even a simple intervention was capable of producing significant reductions in mortality and morbidity.

The largest confirmation of the advantage of the checklist came from the adoption by the Veterans Health Administration (VHA) in the United States. The VHA is the largest integrated healthcare system in the United States with 153 hospitals. The VHA implemented a team-trained program and a checklist implementation in half of their hospitals during a 2-year period from 2006 to 2008, contemporaneous with the WHO study going on internationally. In the 74 facilities where the training program was implemented, there was an 18% reduction in annual mortality rate, which compared with a 7% decrease among 34 facilities that had not yet undergone implementation of the checklist and briefing program [36]. This study differed from the WHO program in that the hospitals that had not yet undergone implementation of the training program served as a viable control group to demonstrate the effectiveness of the intervention. After eventual implementation in all VHA hospitals, the mortality rate had declined similarly in all of them. The VHA program included the use of a checklist as a central component of a preprocedural team briefing, and was associated with educational efforts to enhance team communication and performance. Implementation of the program was also associated with decreased OR delays [37] and improvement in antibiotic administration and deep venous thromboprophylaxis compliance [38].

ADOPTING THE WHO CHECKLIST: BARRIERS APPEAR

Despite the incontrovertible data supporting the positive effects of the checklist-centered preprocedural pause, acceptance and effective implementation was not universal. The surgery department at Vanderbilt University Medical Center used a briefing script and a whiteboard along with Crew Resource Management (CRM) training for their surgical teams, but observed only a 57% compliance with their 62 designated safety steps when directly assessing their results in the OR [39]. Northwestern Memorial Hospital in Chicago (part of Northwestern University) also used 4-hour team training exercises along with a preoperative structured briefing led by the surgeon. Two weeks after the training, 86% of cases included a briefing, which fell to 66% at the 6- to 8-month follow-up, despite improvements in safety attitudes surveys [40]. The SafeSurgery group itself conducted a follow-up on five selected hospitals in the State of Washington, where adoption was first completed statewide in the United States. They found that three of the five hospitals had only "incomplete" implementation 9 to 10 months after introduction of the checklist [41]. They concluded that active leadership, institutional support, and dedicated resources were essential, but that the effectiveness of the checklist was likely to vary with the effectiveness of implementation at a local level.

In an academic atmosphere where authors primarily report their successes, the appearance of these reports (especially one from the original sponsoring group) suggests that there may be even more challenges to universal adoption. What, then, are the barriers to universal effectiveness of checklists?

LIMITATIONS OF CHECKLISTS

The published experiences reflect the experience of the aviation industry. Aviation had been using checklists since 1934, and yet in 1977, 683 people died when two 747 jumbo jets collided on the runway at Tenerife airport in the Canary Islands. Among the significant findings in the investigation was the revelation that junior flight crewmembers realized that they did not have a clear approval for take-off, but were reluctant to challenge the senior captain. Among many changes made after this disaster, one was the push for a cultural change in the industry, to move away from the authoritarian and hierarchical historical structure where decisions of the senior members were not open to question. This produced five evolutions of crew communication training systems, moving from "cockpit resource management" to "crew resource management." Even the later generations of CRM struggled with the challenge of "highly individualistic cultures, such as the United States, [which] stress independence from the group and priority for personal goals" – in other words, the frequency of "cowboys" as they were referred to. Now the "fifth generation" of crew training stresses that CRM is only one tool to engage the entire team in the effort to reduce the risk of inevitable human error [42] and that open communication is essential.

Medicine is undergoing a similar evolution, recognizing that safety is not just about personal achievement and system design, but also about relationships [43]. The traditions of autonomy and "craftsmanship" status of the profession [44] may represent challenges to adopting new safety steps, such as checklists, if the reluctance to question an authority figure (physician, especially surgeon) remains. The "perfectionist" model of medical practice [8] leads physicians to accept an unrealistic burden of responsibility, and a reluctance to ask for or accept help. Unfortunately, it is part of medicine: physicians are trained in an environment that encourages independent work as a cultural expectation and discourages the concept of calling for help [45]. This may be one of the factors that lead 10% of practicing physicians to reject evidenced-based guidelines [46]. Some of these patterns may account for part of the limitations of implementation of safety steps, such as checklists. The newer model of error prevention, where one recognizes that all people are prone to error, and need to be willing to accept the support of groups and peers in helping to avoid error, requires a cultural change.

BARRIER OF HIERARCHY

The challenge of hierarchy and particularly surgical reluctance is mentioned in several reports of attempts to implement checklists. Fourcade and colleagues [47] in France found that "time-honored hierarchy" was a barrier in one-third of cases. Vats and coworkers [48] in the United Kingdom found that "some consultant surgeons were not very enthusiastic" and compliance with the checklist rose slowly to 79% 6 months after implementation. In Canada, Lingard and colleagues [27] found that autonomy remained a barrier in effective briefing and in a few situations led to "mindless and rote" recitation of the checklist by a few physicians who saw the briefing as an exercise "that needs to be completed rather than an opportunity to enhance team communication" [49]. In the United States, Sax and colleagues [50] from Brown University reported success in achieving the checklist with team training, but on the safety questionnaires, a trend toward hierarchical effects remained, with staff less comfortable challenging physicians than nurses or technicians. The cardiovascular surgery group at the Mayo Clinic introduced a checklist that improved OR efficiency, but found in their staff interviews that 35% believed the surgeon's behavior negatively affected team function [51]. Pronovost from Johns Hopkins acknowledged that some of the clinicians in his group resisted adopting their safety interventions [52], and a report in the Harvard Business Review even highlighted the barriers of physician autonomy [53]. All of these observations suggest the need for a cultural change in medicine to support the adoption of safer practices.

ROLE OF CULTURAL CHANGE, TEAM TRAINING

The need for culture change was recognized in some of the earliest attempts to improve OR safety. Zohar and colleagues [54] found limited success with a purely educational program to ensure correct-sited surgery that did not include team training and cultural change. However, Mazzocco and colleagues [55] in the Kaiser Hospital system in the southwestern United States investigated the effect of positive team behaviors on patient outcome. In a review of 300 patients, they found that teams that displayed lower communication and information sharing in the perioperative period were associated with a 4.82 greater odds of adverse outcomes (complications or death) compared with teams with high scores. The implications of this impact of team behaviors on outcome suggest it is important to measure those factors and include assessments in evaluating safety. Several tools have been used, mostly based on the SAQ, which is derived from the aviation experience. Using this tool, several studies have found wide variations in safety cultures. In 2006, Makary and coworkers evaluated surgical staff at 60 hospitals in a Catholic healthcare system. The perception of a "good safety climate" varied from 14% to 100% across the institutions (Fig. 3) [56]. Another aspect of their data, confirmed in other studies, was significant discrepancies in how groups rated each other. Basically, surgeons frequently described teamwork as "good" when their nursing colleagues perceived it as less effective [57]. This suggests that posting a checklist alone may not be as effective a safety tool as team training to improve staff communication and team behaviors.

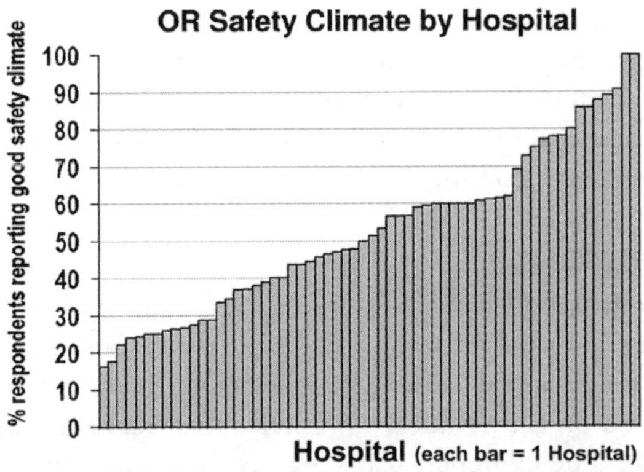

Fig. 3. Safety climate by hospital (each bar represents one hospital). (*From* Makary MA, Sexton JB, Freischlag JA, et al. Patient safety in surgery. Ann Surg 2006;243(5):628–32; with permission.)

THE CHECKLIST AS A STEP TO HELP OVERCOME BARRIERS

This discussion puts the checklist in a broader perspective, not as a single tool to provide safety, but as a framework for a group discussion to enhance communication and team function. Most of the initial efforts of Lingard, Makary, and others started as "briefings," not just checklists, and many of the studies cited here have shown improvements in teamwork scores with the adoption of this combination checklist/briefing. Using the objective checklist as a framework for the discussion may actually "empower nurses and junior-level physicians to insist that those higher in the traditional hierarchy adhere to approved and safe procedures" [5]. Several groups have found that adding the briefing and checklist increase compliance with safety steps [58]. Another advantage is that the addition of a structured briefing produces a de facto CRM training, where each member of the team learns to speak his or her part and participate on an equal footing without official training.

OTHER CHALLENGES OF ADOPTION: TIME AND MONEY, SUSTAINABILITY

Several institutions have incurred expense in terms of time and money to do team training. The original Kaiser briefing involved additional staff at a cost of $50,000 [22]. The VHA implementation was achieved by closing their ORs for a full day for team training. The success in eliminating delays at the University of California San Francisco VHA also required a full day of training out of the OR [37]. The Rotterdam Ophthalmologic Institute in the Netherlands successfully transported their entire staff off-site to experience CRM training in an airline simulator to enhance their team performance [59]. Although many experts agree that such team building is the critical step (in addition to the checklist), resources may not be available in all institutions to provide extensive training and the resources to accurately gauge its outcomes [52].

Another "cost" is the issue of sustainability. Others have found challenges in preserving changes in practices, such as blood transfusion or checklists [60,61]. Each institution must include a program or system to ensure that use of a checklist and briefing is maintained after the initial enthusiasm, and in the face of the inevitable new changes coming yearly in medical care.

FUTURE DIRECTIONS

It is unlikely that the surgical checklist will be replaced. Evidence for the effectiveness of checklists [31] suggests they will find wider applications in medicine. There is good evidence in simulation scenarios that "emergency situation" checklists modeled on the aviation experience may be useful in critical medical situations [62,63]. The evidence also suggests they may find an increasing role in helping clinicians to follow evidence-based pathways more effectively than is currently practiced in the United States.

SUMMARY

Preoperative checklists have been shown to be highly effective in improving compliance with safety steps and reducing perioperative morbidity and mortality. Their effectiveness seems to be enhanced when they are used as a framework for a team briefing that is used to improve communication and promote team behaviors, including empowering junior staff to question more senior authority figures and feeling free to communicate their concerns. It seems such a cultural change is essential to ensure full implementation and sustainability of a preprocedural pause/checklist and to effect significant improvements in patient safety. There also seems to be an increasing role for these cognitive aids in assisting physicians in handling evidence-based pathways and emergency situations.

References

[1] Reason J. Human error: models and management. BMJ 2000;320:768–70.
[2] Reason J. Human error. New York: Cambridge University Press; 1990. p. 234–41.
[3] John Schamel. How the Pilot's Checklist Came About.http://www.atchistory.org/History/checklst.htm. Accessed 5 September, 2012.
[4] Karl R. Briefings, checklists, geese, and surgical safety. Ann Surg Oncol 2010;17:8–11.
[5] Winters BD, Gurses AP, Lehmann H, et al. Clinical review. Checklists: translating evidence into practice. Crit Care 2009;13(6):210.
[6] Boorman DJ. Today's electronic checklists reduce likelihood of crew errors and help prevent mishaps. ICAO J 2001;1:17–22.
[7] Hales B, Terblanche M, Fowler R, et al. Development of medical checklists for improved quality of patient care. Int J Qual Health Care 2008;20(1):22–30.
[8] Leape LL. Error in medicine. JAMA 1994;272:1851–7.
[9] Kohn LL, Corrigan JM, Donaldson MS. To err is human. Washington (DC): Institute of Medicine, National Academy Press; 1999.
[10] Bohnen JM, Lingard L. Error and surgery: can we do better? Can J Surg 2003;46(5):327–9.
[11] Vincent C, Moorthy K, Sarker SK, et al. Systems approaches to surgical quality and safety: from concept to measurement. Ann Surg 2004;239(4):475–82.
[12] March MG, Crowley JJ. An evaluation of anesthesiologists' present checkout methods and the validity of the FDA checklist. Anesthesiology 1991;75(5):724–9.

[13] Arbous MS, Meursing AE, van Kleef JW, et al. Impact of anesthesia management characteristics on severe morbidity and mortality. Anesthesiology 2005;102(2):257–68.
[14] Wolff AM, Taylor SA, McCabe JF. Using checklists and reminders in clinical pathways to improve hospital inpatient care. Med J Aust 2004;181(8):428–31.
[15] Young GB, Frewen T, Barr HW, et al. Checklist for diagnosis of brain death. Can J Neurol Sci 1991;18(1):104.
[16] Schectman JM, Schorling JB, Nadkarni MM, et al. The effect of physician feedback and an action checklist on diabetes care measures. Am J Med Qual 2004;19(5):207–13.
[17] Hall RI, Rocker GM, Murray D. Simple changes can improve conduct of end-of-life care in the intensive care unit. Can J Anaesth 2004;51(6):631–6.
[18] Pronovost P, Berenholtz S, Dorman T, et al. Improving communication in the ICU using daily goals. J Crit Care 2003;18(2):71–5.
[19] O'Grady NP, Alexander M, Dellinger EP, et al. Guidelines for the prevention of intravascular catheter-related infections. MMWR Recomm Rep 2002;51(RR-10):1–29.
[20] Berenholtz SM, Pronovost PJ, Lipsett PA, et al. Eliminating catheter-related bloodstream infections in the intensive care unit. Crit Care Med 2004;32(10):2014–20.
[21] Pronovost P, Needham D, Berenholtz S, et al. An intervention to decrease catheter-related bloodstream infections in the ICU. N Engl J Med 2006;355(26):2725–32.
[22] DeFontes J. Preoperative safety briefing project. Perm J 2004;8:21–7.
[23] Makary MA, Holzmueller CG, Thompson D, et al. Operating room briefings: working on the same page. Jt Comm J Qual Patient Saf 2006;32(6):351–5.
[24] Makary MA, Mukherjee A, Sexton JB, et al. Operating room briefings and wrong-site surgery. J Am Coll Surg 2007;204:236–43.
[25] Nundy S, Mukherjee A, Sexton JB, et al. Impact of preoperative briefings on operating room delays: a preliminary report. Arch Surg 2008;143:1068–72.
[26] Lingard L, Espin S, Rubin B, et al. Getting teams to talk: development and pilot implementation of a checklist to promote interprofessional communication in the OR. Qual Saf Health Care 2005;14(5):340–6.
[27] Lingard L, Regehr G, Orser B, et al. Evaluation of a preoperative checklist and team briefing among surgeons, nurses, and anesthesiologists to reduce failures in communication. Arch Surg 2008;143(1):12–7.
[28] Lingard L, Regehr G, Cartmill C, et al. Evaluation of a preoperative team briefing: a new communication routine results in improved clinical practice. BMJ Qual Saf 2011;20(6):475–82.
[29] WHO, SSSL_Brochure_finalJun08.pdf, WHO.int; http://www.who.int/patientsafety/safesurgery/knowledge_base/SSSL_Brochure_finalJun08.pdf, 2008. Accessed 5 September, 2012.
[30] WHO, Safe Surgery Checklist, WHO.int, http://www.who.int/patientsafety/safesurgery/tools_resources/SSSL_Checklist_finalJun08.pdf, 2008. Accessed 5 September, 2012.
[31] Gawande A. The checklist manifesto. New York: Henry Holt & Co; 2009. p. 114–35.
[32] Haynes AB, Weiser TG, Berry WR, et al, Safe Surgery Saves Lives Study Group. A surgical safety checklist to reduce morbidity and mortality in a global population. N Engl J Med 2009;360:491–9.
[33] Weiser TG, Haynes AB, Dziekan G, et al, Safe Surgery Saves Lives Investigators and Study Group. Effect of a 19-item surgical safety checklist during urgent operations in a global patient population. Ann Surg 2010;251:976–80.
[34] WHO Safe Surgery Saves Lives Newsletter, April, 2010, WHO.int; http://www.safesurg.org/uploads/1/0/9/0/1090835/april_newsletter.pdf. Accessed 5 September, 2012.
[35] de Vries EN, Prins HA, Crolla RM, et al, SURPASS Collaborative Group. Effect of a comprehensive surgical safety system on patient outcomes. N Engl J Med 2010;363:1928–37.
[36] Neily J, Mills PD, Young-Xu Y, et al. Association between implementation of a medical team training program and surgical mortality. JAMA 2010;304:1693–700.

[37] Wolf FA, Way LW, Stewart L. The efficacy of medical team training: improved team performance and decreased operating room delays: a detailed analysis of 4863 cases. Ann Surg 2010;252:477–83.
[38] Paull DE, Mazzia LM, Wood SD, et al. Briefing guide study: preoperative briefing and postoperative debriefing checklists in the Veterans Health Administration medical team-training program. Am J Surg 2010;200(5):620–3.
[39] France DJ, Leming-Lee S, Jackson T, et al. An observational analysis of surgical team compliance with perioperative safety practices after crew resource management training. Am J Surg 2008;195:546–53.
[40] Halverson AL, Andersson JL, Anderson K, et al. Surgical team training: the Northwestern Memorial Hospital experience. Arch Surg 2009;144:107–12.
[41] Conley DM, Singer SJ, Edmondson L, et al. Effective surgical safety checklist implementation. J Am Coll Surg 2011;212:873–9.
[42] Helmreich RL, Merritt AC, Wilhelm JA. The evolution of Crew Resource Management training in commercial aviation. Int J Aviat Psychol 1999;9(1):19–32.
[43] Leape LL. New world of patient safety: 23rd Annual Samuel Jason Mixter lecture. Arch Surg 2009;144(5):394–8.
[44] Amalberti R, Auroy Y, Berwick D, et al. Five system barriers to achieving ultrasafe health care. Ann Intern Med 2005;142:756–64.
[45] Kennedy TJ, Regehr G, Baker GR, et al. It's a cultural expectation. The pressure on medical trainees to work independently in clinical practice. Med Educ 2009;43(7):645–53.
[46] Cabana MD, Rand CS, Powe NR, et al. Why don't physicians follow clinical practice guidelines? A framework for improvement. JAMA 1999;282(15):1458–65.
[47] Fourcade A, Blache JL, Grenier C, et al. Barriers to staff adoption of a surgical safety checklist. BMJ Qual Saf 2012;21(3):191–7.
[48] Vats A, Vincent CA, Nagpal K, et al. Practical challenges of introducing WHO surgical checklist: UK pilot experience. BMJ 2010;340:b5433.
[49] Khoshbin A, Lingard L, Wright JG. Evaluation of preoperative and perioperative operating room briefings at the Hospital for Sick Children. Can J Surg 2009;52:309–15.
[50] Sax HC, Browne P, Mayewski RJ, et al. Can aviation-based team training elicit sustainable behavioral change? Arch Surg 2009;144:1133–7.
[51] ElBardissi AW, Wiegmann DA, Dearani JA, et al. Application of the human factors analysis and classification system methodology to the cardiovascular surgery operating room. Ann Thorac Surg 2007;83:1412–8.
[52] Pronovost PJ, Freischlag JA. Improving teamwork to reduce surgical mortality. JAMA 2010;304(15):1721–2.
[53] Lee TH. Turning doctors into leaders. Harv Bus Rev 2010;88(4):50–8.
[54] Zohar E, Noga Y, Davidson E, et al. Perioperative patient safety: correct patient, correct surgery, correct side. A multifaceted, cross-organizational, interventional study. Anesth Analg 2007;105(2):443–7.
[55] Mazzocco K, Petitti DB, Fong KT, et al. Surgical team behaviors and patient outcomes. Am J Surg 2009;197:678–85.
[56] Makary MA, Sexton JB, Freischlag JA, et al. Patient safety in surgery. Ann Surg 2006;243(5):628–32.
[57] Makary MA, Sexton JB, Freischlag JA, et al. Operating room teamwork among physicians and nurses: teamwork in the eye of the beholder. J Am Coll Surg 2006;202:746–52.
[58] Altpeter T, Luckhardt K, Lewis JN, et al. Expanded surgical time out: a key to real-time data collection and quality improvement. J Am Coll Surg 2007;204(4):527–32.
[59] de Korne DF, van Wijngaarden JD, Hiddema UF, et al. Diffusing aviation innovations in a hospital in The Netherlands. Jt Comm J Qual Patient Saf 2010;36:339–47.
[60] Tobin SN, Campbell DA, Boyce NW. Durability of response to a targeted intervention to modify clinician transfusion practices in a major teaching hospital. Med J Aust 2001;174:445–8.

[61] Johnston G, Ekert L, Pally E. Surgical site signing and "time out": issues of compliance or complacence. J Bone Joint Surg Am 2009;91:2577–80.
[62] Ziewacz JE, Arriaga AF, Bader AM, et al. Crisis checklists for the operating room: development and pilot testing. J Am Coll Surg 2011;213(2):212–7.
[63] Neal JM, Hsiung RL, Mulroy MF, et al. ASRA checklist improves trainee performance during a simulated episode of local anesthetic systemic toxicity. Reg Anesth Pain Med 2012;37(1): 8–15.

Advances in Anesthesia 30 (2012) 171–175

INDEX

Note: Page numbers of article titles are in **boldface** type.

0737-6146/12/$ – see front matter
http://dx.doi.org/10.1016/S0737-6146(12)00028-7

D

U

V

W